The Adult Stroke Patient

A Manual for Evaluation and Treatment of Perceptual and Cognitive Dysfunction

Revised Second Edition

Barbara Zoltan, MA OTR
Ellen Siev, OTR
Brenda Freishtat, OTR

SLACK Incorporated, 6900 Grove Road, Thorofare, NJ 08086-9447

SLACK International Book Distributors

In Canada:
McGraw-Hill Ryerson Limited
330 Progress Avenue
Scarborough, Ontario
M1P 2Z5

In Europe and the United Kingdom:
Quest-Meridien Ltd.
Beckham, Kent
England BR3 3RB

In Australia and New Zealand:
MacLennan & Petty Pty Limited
P.O. Box 425
Artarmon, N.S.W. 2064
Australia

In Asia and India:
PG Publishing Pte Limited.
36 West Coast Road, #02-02
Singapore 0512

In Japan:
Igaku-Shoin, Ltd.
Tokyo International P.O. Box 5063
1-28-36 Hongo, Bunkyo-Ku
Tokyo 113
Japan

Foreign Translation Agent

John Scott & Company
International Publishers' Agency
417-A Pickering Road
Phoenixville, PA 19460
Fax: 215-988-0185

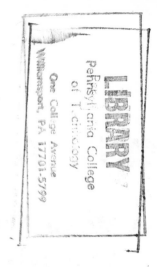

Editor: Cheryl D. Willoughby
Publisher: Harry C. Benson

Printed in the United States of America

Library of Congress Catalog Card Number: 85-50368

ISBN 1-55642-197-4

Published by: SLACK Incorporated
               6900 Grove Road
               Thorofare, NJ 08086-9447

Last digit is print number: 10   9   8   7   6   5   4

Contents

Introduction

In 1976 there were 594,000 people hospitalized for an initial cerebral vascular accident.[200] It is estimated that there are 500,000 new adult victims of cerebral vascular accidents annually in the United States, and that at any given time there are 2 million who have survived strokes.[164] Of those surviving the initial insult, 50 percent will live another five years and 75 percent will be rehabilitated to some degree of independence. Of these new patients, 60 to 70 percent can expect to become ambulatory, although significant functional return of the affected upper extremity is expected in only 30 to 40 percent.

Until recently, rehabilitation focused on restoration of motion and compensation for lost functional skills. Perceptual, visual and cognitive deficits, noted for many years to exist as a result of cerebral vascular accidents, have only recently been acknowledged as a cause of continued confusion and lack of rehabilitation progress in many patients even though motor skills have returned.

Perceptual visual and cognitive deficits have been widely described in the literature, and numerous studies have hypothesized correlations between specific deficits and location of brain damage and have identified deficits that tended to occur simultaneously. However, little has been done to definitively formulate evaluation techniques, to correlate these deficits with functional loss, or to formulate treatment methods.

This manual includes the most useful and most current information pertaining to the occupational therapist's clinical needs in identifying and rehabilitating patients with visual perceptual and cognitive problems. Since it is intended to be a resource book, the material has been documented as closely as possible for future referencing. Before using the enclosed information clinically, the following procedure is suggested.

If it is not possible to read the entire manual, read the initial explanatory notes in Chapter I describing deficits, evaluations, and treatment. Look for the basic differences in deficit descriptions and learn which deficits commonly occur together.

For all tests described, whether standardized or nonstandardized, the student and therapist should practice the evaluations initially on non-brain damaged persons. This will provide experience in test administration and familiarity with normal responses before using patient test results for diagnostic purposes.

Several selected evaluation tools and treatment techniques are listed under each deficit. It behooves the therapist to experiment with various methods in order to find the ones that best suit the needs of both the therapist and the patient.

To enhance the clinical usefulness of this manual, therapists in several occupational therapy departments in this country have been interviewed. The purpose of these interviews was to learn the latest methods for testing and treatment of visual, perceptual, and cognitive problems in the adult patient who has sustained a cerebral vascular accident and to determine the most common problems in treating such patients. It is hoped that this material will provide a concise, useful tool for evaluating and treating these deficits in these patients while raising questions for further research in this area.

Acknowledgments

For Time and Ideas

Dottie Ecker, M.A., O.T.R., F.A.O.T.A.,
and Liane Michael, M.A., C.C.S.P.

For Clerical Support

The Northern California Regional Spinal Injury System, Grant G008435010, Project 128EH40013, from the Rehabilitation Services Administration, U.S. Department of Education, Washington, D.C.

CHAPTER I

Explanations for Use of This Manual

The perceptual problems following adult cerebral vascular accident (CVA) victims have been divided into the following categories for clarity in this manual: body image and body scheme difficulties (Chapter IV), spatial relations problems (Chapter V), apraxias (Chapter III), and agnosias (Chapter VI).

The visual problems following a CVA have been divided into visual attention, oculomotor skills (pursuits and saccades), visual fields, and visual neglect and are covered in Chapter II. The cognitive portion has been divided into attention, memory, initiation, planning, insight, mental flexibility, problem solving, and acalculia. Cognitive deficits are covered in Chapter VIII. It should be noted that although described separately, several deficits are frequently interrelated and occur together. Information about aphasia (Chapter VII) is included in this manual, not only because it is related to specific perceptual deficits, mainly body scheme, apraxias, and agnosias, but also because aphasia often masks perceptual problems and thus complicates evaluation and treatment. Age-related deficits, vision, sensory loss, environment, and motor deficits are also described because they, too, may complicate perceptual and cognitive deficits.

Each chapter concerned with an area of vision, perception or cognition is subdivided into sections for specific deficits, each containing information about description, lesion site information, evaluation, and treatment for that deficit. This format is used repeatedly throughout Chapters II through VIII. Even though lesion site information is provided, it should be noted that there is great variability in the human brain from one individual to another. Thus, two patients with brain lesions in exactly the same location may have different resultant deficits. In addition, it must be remembered that the brain functions as a whole and that damage to one part influences more than just the perceptual or cognitive symptom identified for that particular site.

Deficit Descriptions

In the average adult, visual, perceptual and cognitive skills are highly developed. Following a cerebral vascular accident, certain perceptual or cognitive deficits may result, probably from brain damage at the cortical integrative level for sensory input.[48] Certain deficits occur as a result of only right- or left-sided brain lesions; others may occur as a result of a lesion in either hemisphere.

Following each deficit description, the probable site of the lesion that causes the deficit is stated.

The remainder of this chapter will provide the necessary background data to enable the reader to use the manual more effectively.

Deficit Evaluation

In Chapters II through VIII, immediately following the descriptions of each deficit, the visual perceptual or cognitive tests used to evaluate that deficit in the adult brain damaged patient are described. Because most of these tests have not been validated, several tests are listed under each deficit. The authors believe that the patient's performance on a minimum of at least two tests should be considered in attempting to evaluate his problem. However, the reader is cautioned that because of the time/cost ratio involved in evaluation procedures, it is not always possible or necessary to test the patient for every deficit described.

Test Reliability and Validity

Before describing specific evaluations, a few precautions for interpreting test results are in order. Some of the tests presented in this text are subjective rather than objective. Objective tests are defined as those in which one examiner, following directions, will score a given performance of a test in the same way as another examiner. In subjective tests, the examiner observes the patient's performance of a given test item and evaluates the performance according to his own judgment of the quality of the response. The examiner observes not only whether a patient can or cannot perform the task but also how well he performs it. Although numbers can be assigned in the scoring of subjective tests, in the tests described in this manual, the scores are usually descriptive. A score of intact, impaired, severely impaired, or absent is assigned. In other words, on a subjective test, the results are evaluated qualitatively; on an objective test, they are evaluated quantitatively (although analysis of qualitative performance will provide additional data).

A test's reliability refers to its consistency and accuracy. Reliability can be measured in several ways. One way is to administer a test to an individual several times. If the score is approximately the same over repeated examinations, the test-retest reliability is said to be good. By repeating this procedure with a large group of people, one can perform a statistical analysis and derive a coefficient of correlation (r) for the test. A test's test-retest correlation (r) can range from 0 to 1.0. The higher the r, the better the test-retest reliability. If a test has a test-retest correlation of 0.60 or higher, it is considered fairly reliable. One should be sure that a test has a fairly high test-retest correlation if one intends to use the test as a measure of improvement following treatment.

Scorer or inter-rater response is another method of measuring a test's reliability. Here two or more examiners score a set of tests and their results are compared. The closer the sets of scores are to each other, the better the test's scorer reliability. Again, the range of the coefficient of correlation (r) is from 0 to 1.0, and the closer it is to 1.0, the better. The results of tests of reliability are usually found in a test's manual.

Unless the criteria for making the judgment for score assignment is explicit on a subjective test, the scorer reliability of the test is likely to be low. Therefore, it is difficult to compare results between patients or between testings of the same patient if the tests are scored by different examiners. However, since anyone giving an objective test should get the same results as anyone else, the scorer reliability is likely to be high. It still may not be a reliable or consistent test; its test-retest reliability may be low.

Only a few of the objective visual, perceptual or cognitive tests have been standardized for adult populations, although some have been standardized for children. A standardized test is defined as any test that has been administered to a large sample of the population one wishes to test so that the examiner knows how the average person in this population scores on this test. When tests have not been standardized, interpretation of scores is tenuous, since there are no norms for comparison. In such instances it is suggested that if one is unfamiliar with the test and with how the normal adult will perform, it should first be administered to several normal adults, preferably of the same age, sex, and occupational or educational level as the patient. In this way one can develop skill in test administration and gain some idea of how well a normal adult should score on the test.

The validity of many of these tests has not been examined. A test's validity refers to how well the test measures what it purports to measure. There are several types of validity. One type, content validity, describes how well the test represents the total universe of the content of the property being measured. Deciding the degree to which it does this is, basically, a matter of judgment. However, other types of validity can be measured by statistical analysis. The results of such tests are usually found in a test's manual. Although many of the tests reported here have content validity, in our judgment their total validity has not been statistically established. For this reason a low score on any one test is not conclusive evidence that the patient has that particular deficit. A low score on one test should signal the need for follow-up with a series of similar tests.

Very few studies have been done to correlate results of tests of perception and cognition with actual functional abilities and disabilities. This is part of examining the test's validity. For example, an adult patient may do very poorly on *Ayres' Figure-Ground Test* yet show no observable functional deficit in that area. Those perceptual or cognitive tests that have been shown to correlate with functional performance will be specified when each specific deficit is described. The problem of lack of research to correlate test scores and functional performance has led some occupational therapists to rely solely on functional tests, e.g., can a patient dress himself, rather than on formal perceptual or cognitive tests. The problem that functional tests present is that one cannot always discern why the patient is having trouble doing the task. One can hypothesize reasons and then test them with the more discrete formal perceptual tests. In this way a combination of functional and perceptual or cognitive tasks can be most useful.

Administration of Tests

In actually administering the tests described in the following chapters, one should be aware of several additional problems. First, none of these tests measure completely discrete functions. They may emphasize one main function, but most overlap into other areas. To use these tests with greater validity, one must first rule out other deficits the patient may have. For example, in testing tactile agnosia, the inability to recognize objects by touch although sensation is intact, one must first test to be sure that the patient has normal tactile sensation. Throughout the test descriptions, under the heading "To Improve Validity," we will list those deficits that should be tested first to rule out their interference with the patient's performance on the test being described. Unfortunately, other deficits may be an inherent part of the test and thus be impossible to rule out. For example, a right hemiplegic patient and a left hemiplegic patient may perform equally poorly on *Benton's Three-Dimensional Constructional Praxis Test* but for entirely different reasons. The right hemiplegic tends to have trouble initiating or carrying through the construction, which is more an execution problem; the left hemiplegic tends to pick up and move blocks around randomly, which is more a spatial relations problem.[186] Therefore, the examiner must be aware of the different causes of poor performance on a given test and look closely at the qualitative performance by the patient for clues to the reason for his failure.

Second, all the tests require comprehension of the directions, and some require verbal responses. Thus their use with aphasic patients must take this into account. These tests may not be valid for aphasics; they may measure language rather than perceptual or cognitive skills.

Third, many of the tests require some motor act as part of the response. Patients should first be tested for apraxia and lack of motor control to rule out problems in the areas in the tests at which a motor response is required.

Fourth, although the patient appears to be mentally alert, he may do poorly on the tests because he is inattentive or easily distracted. This may be the result of brain damage. According to Luria,[151] lesions in the frontal lobe affect a patient's ability to form intentions or goals, to attend and concentrate. The patient may be inattentive because the task is too abstract for him. Hague[114] showed that left hemiplegics have a definite impairment of complex abstract behavior and should be tested on the concrete level. Or a patient may have a very short immediate visual memory, making it difficult for him to attend to the task.[53,229] These and other cognitive deficits are covered in Chapter VIII.

Vision is also a factor in many of these tests. Often patients who have sustained a stroke are old and have poor eyesight that is not always corrected well by their glasses. This should be checked before administering tests in which visual acuity is important. Information about aging, vision, and visual evaluation and treatment are covered in detail in Chapters II, VII, and IX.

A patient's prestroke intelligence, perceptual cognitive skills, and educational and cultural background can also affect his performance. For example, if a patient was developmentally delayed before his stroke, he will have difficulty with some abstract concepts in the tests even if he has no perceptual or cognitive problems as a result of the stroke. Or if his background is such that he never learned to write or draw, paper and pencil tests may not be valid. Or if, for various reasons, he never developed his perceptual or cognitive skills to their fullest capacity, low scores on the tests would not necessarily be the result of his stroke.

Lastly, one may get poor results because the patient reacts negatively to this type of testing. He may find the tasks childish and refuse to do them. Or he may think that they are intelligence tests and become very anxious about his performance. For this reason one must be careful in explaining the purpose of all tests.

Because of the nature of these tests, it is recommended that one use a quiet area with few distractions to test the patient and limit testing to short periods each day.

Test Scoring

If the test has been standardized, it is important to administer it exactly according to the accompanying directions in order to use the test's norms.

Three categories of tests are examined in this manual. They are:
1. Standardized—scored objectively, standardized with adults.
2. Nonstandardized—scored objectively, not standardized with adults.
3. Subjective—scored subjectively, not standardized.

In scoring subjective and nonstandardized tests, a patient's performance is usually labeled intact, impaired, severely impaired, or absent. An intact performance is defined as the way a normal adult would perform on the test. A severely impaired/absent performance is defined as one in which the patient is making many errors, taking longer than normal to do the test, or having trouble completing the test. An impaired performance is between a severely impaired and an intact performance. The patient completes the test but makes one or two errors or does not perform the task quite correctly. For example, on the *Block Bridges Test* for spatial relations, in which the patient is asked to copy and build a three-block bridge, a five-block bridge, and then a seven-block bridge, an intact performance would consist of all bridges being built correctly. An impaired performance would consist of one or two blocks being omitted, out of place, or rotated. A severely impaired performance would consist of the bridges being severely out of proportion or unrecognizable or the patient being unable to do the task.

In the following chapters, an intact performance will be described on those tests scored subjectively or nonstandardized. If the patient's performance is not intact, the labeling of his performance as "impaired" or "severely impaired" will at times be left up to the examiner, since the differences between the two is one of degree of impairment.

When some tests are used to evaluate more than one deficit, a description of an impaired performance will be included to distinguish qualitative differences of performance between patients with different deficits. For example, the *Copy Flower, House Test,* in which the patient is asked to copy a drawing of a house and a flower, is used to test for both unilateral neglect and constructional apraxia. In order to differentiate between the two deficits when the test is examined during evaluations for unilateral neglect, a description of how a patient with unilateral neglect would perform is included.

Treatment of Deficit

In the following chapters, specific suggestions for treatment will be listed under the descriptions of each deficit. These suggestions come from a review of the literature and interview with registered occupational therapists. The suggestions are not proven formulas. They should be adapted and added to as experience and patient needs warrant. Therapists feel that treatment is most beneficial to the patient if it is done on a daily basis.

The approaches to the treatment of perceptual problems in adult hemiplegics will be presented. They are:
1. Sensory integrative approach.
2. Transfer of training approach.
3. Functional approach.
4. Neurodevelopmental approach.

In addition, the cognitive portion of the book contains a section on the influence or use of environment and computers in cognitive rehabilitation.

Sensory Integrative Approach

The sensory integrative approach is used most often by occupational therapists when treating perceptual, cognitive, and behavioral problems in children. The sensory integrative model for treatment is based on neurophysiological and developmental principles, and can be defined as the organization of sensation for use by the individual.[12] Integration converts our initial sensations into meaningful perceptions. Spatial organization, for example, is based on the integration of an assortment of visual, auditory, and kinesthetic cues.[12] Sensory motor integration can occur at all levels of the central nervous system, extending from the spinal cord to the cerebral cortex.[12]

Sensory integration occurs during an adaptive response.[13] The adaptive response is both goal directed and purposeful. During sensory integrative therapy the therapist provides and controls sensory input, especially the input from the vestibular system, muscles, joints, and skin. This controlled sensory stimulation is then followed by an adaptive response by the patient, which will integrate those sensations provided and controlled by the therapist. For more detailed information about sensory integration theory, evaluation, and treatment principles, the reader is referred to references 12 and 13.

Although originally developed for use with children, there is increased interest on the part of occupational therapists in the use of sensory integrative therapy with brain damaged adults. Justification for its use with stroke patients is based on concepts and documented studies in three related areas: aging, the effect of environment on central nervous system functioning and brain plasticity.

The majority of the stroke population are 60 years old or older.[175] One study indicated that 81 percent of the stroke population were 65 to 74 years old and that 92.5 percent were between 75 and 84.[72] It is documented that the well, elderly individual experiences changes in all sensory systems, perception, and intellectual functioning. These changes are described in detail in the section, "The Relationship of Age to Perceptual and Cognitive Evaluation and Treatment," in Chapter IX.

The most relevant changes relative to the elderly (well or brain damaged) and the application of sensory integration are those of the primary sensory systems and the vestibular system. Recent research indicates that there is a decrease in the quantity and diameter of vestibular nerves in the elderly, as well as decreased vestibular reflexes.[135] Age related changes in the sensory components of the central nervous system can result in impaired processing of both the internal and the external environments.[179] Memory loss, one of the most devastating impairments experienced by the elderly, has been linked with modality specific sensory memory.[179] Ordy et al. state, ". . . convergent polysensory information processing in multimodal sensory integration centers within the cerebral cortex and limbic system may play a critical role in the short-term memory impairment of the elderly."[179]

It is well documented that elderly patients lose the ability to adapt effectively to the environment and that autonomic nervous system changes decrease their ability to make adaptive responses. In addition, the elderly experience increasing sensory isolation, which can in turn lead to functional and structural changes in vital sensory links that guide and facilitate adaptation and behavior.[179]

Figure 1-1 summarizes normal sensory integrative functioning and that of

**Figure 1-1. Summary of Normal Sensory Integrative Function and
That of the Elderly Individual**

Normal	Elderly (Well or Brain Damaged)
Sensory stimulation from the environment	Sensory stimulation from the environment
↓	↓
Normal sensory registration and processing	Abnormal sensory registration and processing due to impaired primary sensory systems (i.e., visual, auditory, tactile, olfactory, and gustatory)
↓	↓
Normal sensory integration and interpretation	Abnormal sensory integration and interpretation due to impaired primary sensory systems *and* impaired autonomic, proprioceptive, and vestibular systems
↓	↓
Appropriate functional adaptive response	Poor and inappropriate adaptive response due to impaired primary sensory systems, impaired autonomic, proprioceptive, and vestibular systems *and* age or disability related mobility impairment

the elderly individual. The sensory integrative dysfunction present in the elderly is similar to that in the learning disabled child. It can be hypothesized that some sensory integrative techniques successfully utilized with the learning disabled child also can be effective with the well or brain damaged elderly with similar dysfunction.

The second factor to consider when relating sensory integration and the adult patient is the environment. As previously noted, a major theoretical construct of sensory integration is the necessity for sensory stimulation from the environment for normal functioning. The need for environmental stimulation is emphasized when one considers the results of environmental deprivation. Studies of institutionalized geriatric patients indicated a decrease in the quality of verbalization, difficulties in directed thinking and concentration, drifting of thought, disorientation in time, and complaints of restlessness.[204]

A sensory deprivation study of normal adults indicated that the subjects exhibited a general disorganization of brain function similar to that produced by anoxia or brain tumors.[216]

Although the patient who has sustained a stroke is not in a sensory deprived environment, the limitations caused by the stroke result in the same situation as that of a sensory deprived environment. When an individual suffers from a stroke or any disabling disease, that individual's mobility will be limited. This limitation in mobility in turn prevents the individual from receiving adequate tactile proprioceptive and kinesthetic stimulation. This reduced stimulation has been postulated as the cause of lower mental functioning.[204]

Given the identified need for sensory stimulation from the environment and the stroke patient's mobility deficits, which result in limited access to the environment, controlled sensory stimulation is indicated as a primary treatment approach to facilitate patient functioning.

The final factor to consider in applying sensory integrative techniques to adults is brain plasticity. Brain plasticity refers to the adaptive capacities of the central nervous system. It involves the brain's ability to create functional and structural changes when necessary to increase function.[196] Some researchers state that plasticity is accomplished by collateral axonal sprouting, which occurs after brain damage and serves to take over the function of the damaged area.[15,103] The patient with brain damage therefore learns to substitute alternative mechanisms for those he has lost.

It is well documented that the child's normal development involving continuing environmental interaction causes functional and structural brain changes, which in turn allow the child to deal more effectively with the environment. This is accomplished because the brain is considered "plastic" or malleable. Sensory integrative therapy utilizing the concept of plasticity is based on the premise that directed environmental interaction with the learning disabled child can result in functional neurological changes. Considerable research in this field has supported this premise.

The concept of brain plasticity in mature adults is controversial. Some professionals believe that there is little or no potential for plasticity in the adult brain. Other professionals believe that there is sufficient potential for plasticity in the adult brain to respond to therapeutic intervention. These professionals believe that regardless of the age of the individual, the central nervous system is dynamic and ever-changing.[91] They believe that there is evidence of some type of plasticity, because functional recovery does occur in brain damaged adults, even when the lesion is massive and the patient elderly.[144] Several animal research studies indicate brain plasticity and the potential for the external environment to influence neuroanatomical structures, even in adult organisms.[82,200] Animal research studies have also indicated that an enriched or normal environment slows down and sometimes prevents the decrease in neural functions associated with age.[13] If one believes that brain plasticity does exist in adults, controlled sensory stimulation, followed by adaptive environmental interaction, is indicated as a primary treatment approach.

Although described separately, the concepts pertaining to age, environment, and plasticity are related. The elderly patient suffers losses in all sensory systems, in the vestibular and autonomic nervous systems, and in mobility that results in poor sensory processing and integration. The remediation of the deficits previously described involves concepts related to environment, that is, providing an enriched environment through controlled sensory stimulation. A major underlying concept related to the success in providing this enriched environment is the potential for brain plasticity. Through the brain's potential for plasticity, the elderly individual is able to register and process sensory stimulation from the environment, undergo functional neurological changes related to this stimulation, and subsequently carry out an adaptive response.

Although the theoretical constructs described appear sound, there remains a paucity of documented studies substantiating the use of sensory integration therapy with the adult brain damaged patient. Modification of the approach has been used with geriatric, blind, and hemiplegic adults and is subsequently described.

Baker-Nobles and Bink provided sensory integration therapy to blind adults.[18] They hypothesized that sensory integration problems were responsible for the learning problems, postural problems, and self-stimulating behaviors present in the blind individual. They utilized bolsters, net swings, scooterboards, vibration, rubbing, rolling, tilt boards, obstacle courses, and the like as modes of treatment. The results of their study indicated that the sensory integrative therapy provided caused improvement in equilibrium reactions, postural security, bilateral integration, and tolerance of movement in the subjects of the study.

Fox found that by providing tactile stimulation and deep pressure to the hands of her hemiplegic patients, she could significantly increase their scores on finger localization and morphognosia tests.[93] Fiebert and Brown, in a study of 10 participants and 10 control subjects, provided vestibular stimulation (spinning) to 10 right, left, and bilateral stroke patients aged 56 to 84.[91] These investigators found that the subjects who received the vestibular stimulation showed greater improvement in ambulation than the control patients who did not receive the stimulation.

Results of the few studies presented are far from conclusive. A great deal of substantive controlled research is indicated before sensory integration therapy with brain damaged adults can be completely endorsed.

Before concluding this section, the subject of precautions needs to be addressed. Providing sensory integration therapy and, more specifically, vestibular stimulation to the brain damaged adult can cause nausea, fatigue, dizziness, changes in blood pressure, seizures, and abnormal associated reactions.[248] Measurements of blood pressure and other vital signs should be taken before, during, and after (for up to 24 hours) vestibular stimulation has been provided. The planned initiation of a new technique such as spinning should be communicated to all medical and allied health professionals caring for the patient so that potential problems can be monitored around the clock. Finally, it cannot be stressed enough that the beginning therapist should not attempt to incorporate strong vestibular stimulation, such as rotatory stimulation, into the treatment program unless it is done under the direct supervision of an experienced therapist.

Transfer of Training Approach

The basic assumption of this approach is that practice in a particular perceptual task will affect the patient's performance on similar perceptual tasks.[68] For example, if the patient has a spatial relations problem, such as dressing apraxia, one might have him practice with parquetry blocks in the hope that he will improve functionally in other areas involving spatial relations, such as dressing. This approach is used by Frostig[98] in treating perceptual-motor problems in children. Although this is the type of treatment generally used in the clinic today, some therapists believe that the tasks do not transfer and that using them will only result in developing meaningless splinter skills.

The research is not clear about the efficacy of this approach. Mary Taylor[222] completed a two-year study with adult left hemiplegics using a combination of sensory integrative and transfer of training approaches with her experimental group and standard gross motor training with her control group. In the end, her two groups did not differ significantly on a 40-item ADL (activites of daily living) scale, and she rejected her hypothesis that receiving perceptual-cognitive-motor-function (PCMF) treatment would effect more improvement in ADL than standard treatment. However, in examining the treatment used with her control group, it was observed that they received practice in such spatial relations tasks as parquetry blocks, pegboards, and erector set model-building, practice and verbal instructions in dressing, and kinesthetic and proprioceptive stimulation in their gross motor activites. Therefore, the "controlled" nature of her experiment is in doubt.

Leonard Diller[84] reported a study involving both left and right hemiplegics. The experimental group received, in addition to routine rehabilitation therapies, 10 one-hour training sessions in copying block designs, adapted from the block design test on the WAIS. Diller used a hierarchy of cues, systematically decreasing the level of the cue, until the subject could copy the design unaided. The control group received standard rehabilitation therapies. Not only did the experimental group do better on the block design test in post-testing, but they significantly improved ($p < 0.025$) in five areas in occupational therapy as judged from occupational therapy progress notes by nonpartisan judges. The five areas were (1) the patient's attitude and mood, (2) consistency and attention, (3) degree of assistance required in self-care activities, (4) proficiency in eye-hand coordination, and (5) special problems, e.g., compensation for unilateral inattention.

Anderson and Choy[3] recommend exercises in copying block designs and matchstick designs for improvement in spatial concepts though they give no data to support this recommendation.

Helene Goldman[107] reported improved perception of double simultaneous stimulation in both right and left hemiplegics following seven training sessions in practicing discriminating double simultaneous stimulation. Her sample was divided randomly into two groups: One group receiving training for the first two weeks and no training for the second two weeks, followed by a post-test, and in the second group the previously mentioned procedure was reversed. At the end of four weeks both groups showed improvement. The study does not report whether there were any functional gains accompanying the improvement in double simultaneous stimulation perception.

Because the research in this area is so sparse, one must await further research for the definitive answer as to the efficacy of this treatment approach.

Functional Approach

The functional approach is the repetitive practice of particular tasks, usually activities of daily living tasks, which will make the patient more independent in meeting his basic needs. Its emphasis is on treating the symptom rather than the cause of the problem.

For example, a patient who has spatial relations and body image problems will have trouble dressing himself. By setting up a routine for the patient, teaching him cognitive cues, and diligently practicing dressing, the patient may learn to dress himself. But he still will have spatial relations and body image problems in other areas of daily living.

In treating children with cerebral palsy, therapists often teach a child dressing and feeding, even though he is not ready for it developmentally. They do so because it would be better for the child's social and emotional development if he could do these things himself. The same idea is even more true for adults with cerebral vascular accidents. They have suffered a physical disability with a huge emotional and social impact. The sooner they can be independent in self-care, the better will be their social and emotional well-being.

The functional approach to treatment is the one most favored in the clinic, according to a survey of five occupational therapy departments in rehabilitation hospitals in the Boston area.[250-253] The occupational therapists emphasize "functional treatment" and, for the most part, do not use perceptual training per se and do not believe that it helps except to develop splinter skills. Since the patient is usually in the hospital for a limited time (30 to 90 days), it is believed that functional training is much more practical and more understandable to the patient. Patients often object to abstract perceptual or cognitive training, finding it childish, degrading, and not relevant to their problems. Dressing and kitchen activities are more concrete tasks and ones that the patient can better understand. A note of warning: only pragmatic experience, not research, has shown its efficacy.

The functional approach can be divided into two categories, compensation and adaptation:

Compensation. In the compensation approach, the patient is made aware of his problem and then taught to compensate or make allowance for it. For example, if the patient neglects one-half of space because of unilateral neglect, one would teach him to turn his head or scan with his eyes to the affected side. Or if he had dressing apraxia, one would practice a particular dressing pattern with him daily.

Adaptation. Adaptation usually goes along with compensation. In this approach, one makes changes in or adapts the environment of the patient to compensate for his symptoms. For example, if he tends to neglect one-half of space, one would put all his food and utensils on his unaffected side to be sure that he sees it all. Or if he had figure-ground problems, one would try to unclutter his environment to make it easier for him to find objects. Or if he had topographical disorientation, one would mark the route he must follow every day. Or if he had dressing apraxia, one would color code his clothing for "left" and "right" or "inside" and "outside." Informing the patient's family about his problems so that they can make allowances for them, instead of thinking that the patient is stubborn or crazy, is a more subtle form of adaptation. Adapting the patient's "human" rather than his "nonhuman" environment is of major importance in many ways.

This discussion presents a variety of ways in which one can approach the problem of treating patients with perceptual or cognitive problems. Patients who have had cerebral vascular accidents may improve spontaneously, especially within the first three to six months after a stroke. Therefore, it is difficult to ascertain whether the improvement is the result of the patient's spontaneous improvement or the treatment. In any case, the therapist should evaluate the patient carefully and choose the treatment or combination of treatments believed to be most compatible with the patient and his problems. It is then necessary to continuously re-evaluate the patient to determine the efficacy of the chosen treatment approach with this particular patient. Much research is still needed in the area of perceptual and cognitive problems and their treatment so that choice of treatment can be based on fact rather than fancy.

Effect of Neurodevelopmental Treatment on Perception

Perception is developed and refined as the result of an infant's initial movements and kinesthetic awareness.[136] Initial movements are bilaterally symmetrical and do not include a right-left component. It is through continued motor exploration that the child develops an internal awareness of two sides of the body and their difference (laterality). Through continued development and the use of postural mechanisms, the child develops a sense of directionality. The constant orientation of the body to the external environment, provided by postural mechanisms, enables the child to project his internal laterality into external space. The child develops a stable image of his own body, which in turn acts as a reliable and consistent point of origin for future perceptual responses.[136]

The patient who has sustained a stroke will have abnormal changes in postural mechanisms. Owing to a release of abnormal postural reflex mechanisms, spasticity results and leads in turn to an exaggerated static function rather than normal dynamic postural control.[36] In addition, paralysis and visual and sensory losses cause the patient to lose his sense of laterality as well as his sense of directionality.

The neurodevelopmental treatment approach to the recovery of motor function following a stroke works specifically to inhibit abnormal reflex mechanisms and facilitate normal movement.[36] Tactile and kinesthetic stimulation through handling and movement is provided to encourage contact between the individual and the environment.[76] The patient is taught to move normally in all functional tasks. The ultimate goal is to teach the patient how to control his own movements automatically without the aid of the therapist.[170] The therapist works toward the development of a variety of postural sets that make movements easy and automatic.[36] This in turn makes possible the redevelopment of a normal body scheme, leading in turn to improvement in higher level visual discrimination skills.

The use of the neurodevelopmental treatment approach is recommended not only as an effective means of restoring normal motor function, but also as a means of restoring a normal body scheme that ultimately assists in restoring higher level visual perceptual skills. Examples of the use of neurodevelopmental treatment are described in the sections related to body scheme disorders.

CHAPTER II

Gross Visual Skills Deficits

The first area of deficits to be discussed can be classified as gross visual skills. Vision is an important component or prerequisite to perception and cognition. It is not the occupational therapist's role to perform an extensive eye examination. It is, however, his responsibility to obtain from the physician the necessary information pertaining to the patient's vision.

The clinical evaluation of gross visual skills is within the occupational therapist's role. Evaluation is essential to the interpretation of perceptual and cognitive deficits and should therefore be assessed at the beginning of perceptual testing. Included in the evaluation of gross visual skills are visual attention, oculomotor skills (visual scanning and saccadic eye movements), visual fields, and visual neglect.

Visual Attention

The ability to visually attend is present in elementary form at birth and matures by four weeks.[120] For the normal adult, visual fixation is a voluntary act. The normal adult has no difficulty in selecting objects within his environment and focusing his gaze upon them.[87]

The adult patient who has sustained a stroke may have difficulty in visually attending to objects within the environment. The deficit may be an inability to obtain fixation or the inability to sustain it. It may be associated with or occur separately from spatial or body neglect or inattention.

Lesion site: frontal lobe.[243]

Evaluation of Visual Attention

TEST NO. 1: Attending on Command*,[247]

Procedure: The therapist holds an orange rubber ball on the end of a dowel approximately 18 inches in front of the patient at eye level without moving it. Record in seconds how long the patient can attend to the ball.

Directions: "Keep your eyes on the ball until I tell you to stop." (Additional verbal cues can be given.)

Observe whether the patient locates the object with efficiency and attends to it for any length of time (should be at least 20 seconds). Note whether there is good eye convergence or a divergent gaze.

Scoring:

2—Absent, unable to focus on object.

1—Impaired, can focus but unable to attend for 20 seconds.

0—Intact, can visually attend to the object for at least 20 seconds.

To improve validity, rule out aphasia as a cause of poor performance.

Reliability: This test has established inter-rater reliability (r=0.86) with the adult head trauma patient.[23]

---

* Reproduced with permission from Santa Clara Valley Medical Center, San Jose, California.

Treatment for Visual Attention Deficits

1. In an attempt to utilize subcortical mechanisms believed to be associated with the development of visual attention, utilize a multi-modality approach, and associate sensory input with adaptive motor response, have the patient perform activities such as the following:
   a. Alternately roll to the left/right with hands clasped, and hit a suspended ball that the therapist is holding. (Accurate performance of this task requires visual attention.)
   b. Same as the foregoing but in addition requiring the patient to call out several numbers or letters that have been taped to the ball.[249]
   c. Any gross motor bilateral or unilateral activity involving reaching, knocking down, or locating objects within the environment.
   d. Provide verbal, tactile, kinesthetic, and proprioceptive cuing as appropriate during any visual attention activities. For example, turn the patient's head, or passively move the patient's arm toward the desired object.
2. Applying the concept that the environment can affect performance, treat the inattentive patient in a quiet, nondistracting environment, and limit the objects to which the patient must visually attend.
3. Believing that improvement in one task will transfer to similar tasks, utilize any visual perceptual or perceptual-motor task that requires visual attention to complete.
4. Some clinicians advocate the use of computer games or systems, such as the Controlled Reader, as a means of developing visual attention.

Oculomotor Skills

Visual Scanning (Ocular Pursuits)

Visual scanning is a perceptual skill that is crucial to the efficient processing of visual information.[159] Oculomotor deficits are common after brain damage and can vary depending on the size and location of the lesion.[184] A common defect in visual behavior following right-sided brain damage is difficulty in scanning visual space.[85] Deficits can severely impair the patient's ability to effectively scan his environment and in turn can devastate him functionally.

Lesion site: Figure 2-1 summarizes some visual scanning deficits and associated lesion sites.

Figure 2-1. Visual Scanning (Ocular Pursuits) Deficits and Associated Lesion Sites

Deficit	Lesion Site
Decreased conjugate eye movements	Frontal or occipital lobes
Inability to move the eyes in the horizontal and vertical planes on command	Bilateral basal ganglia
Decreased contralateral horizontal gaze	Large lesion of either hemisphere
Decreased conjugate convergence	Upper part of midbrain
Ocular disorders in all planes, i.e., partial paralysis of gaze in horizontal oblique, rotatory or vertical direction; a variety of types of nystagmus	Brain stem

Evaluation of Visual Scanning (Ocular Pursuits)

TEST NO. 1: Direction of Gaze[59]
Description: All six muscles that move each eye (the four rectus muscles—superior and inferior, lateral and medial—and the two oblique muscles—superior and inferior) are tested. The therapist asks the patient to "look first to one side and then to the other . . . to test the medial and lateral rectus muscles. While looking to the one side, the subject is instructed to look up and down; in this position, the adducted eye is elevated by the superior rectus muscle and depressed by the inferior muscle. The abducted eye is elevated by the inferior oblique muscle."[59]

Repeat the procedure with the opposite side to test the opposite muscles.
Scoring: nonstandardized.
Intact: The patient is able to direct his gaze in all directions as requested.
Impaired: The patient is unable to direct his gaze in one or more directions requested. (Specify which movements are impaired.)
Unable to perform: The patient is unable to direct his gaze in any directions as requested.
To improve validity, rule out aphasia and poor visual attentiveness as causes of poor performance.

TEST NO. 2: Ocular Pursuits*[,247]

Description: The therapist moves the orange rubber ball on the end of a dowel back and forth approximately 18 inches in front of the patient's eyes at eye level. The object is moved two or three times slowly in each direction in this order: horizontally, vertically, diagonally (right to left and left to right), clockwise, and counterclockwise.

Directions: "Follow this ball with your eyes in the direction I move it. Move only your eyes and not your head."

Observe for short visual attention span, abnormal jerky eye movements, and excessive head movement. Observe whether the patient loses track of the object or cannot follow in a smooth pursuit. Note: Nystagmus, particularly at the end of eye movement range or at midline. Again note convergence of eye gaze, difficulty in crossing midline, overshooting, and whether a full range of motion of eye movement is present.

Scoring:

2—Absent, unable to track a moving object.

1—Impaired, has difficulty tracking a moving object in any or all directions.

0—Intact, eyes smoothly follow in all directions.

To improve validity, rule out aphasia and poor visual attentiveness as causes of poor performance.

Reliability: This test has established inter-rater reliability (r=1.0) with a sample of adult patients sustaining head trauma.[23]

Treatment for Visual Scanning Deficits

The following four training principles have been shown to be useful in visual scanning retraining:[85,187]

1. Anchoring or cuing the patient where to begin the visual search. For example, a red tape or marker can be placed to the left at the beginning of all lines to be read or scanned.

2. Pacing or cuing the patient about the speed of his response. This will help control impulsive or erratic scanning and establish an appropriate scanning rate. Slowing the patient down can be accomplished simply by having him call out each number or letter as it appears or by placing a sticker under each one that is called out.[187]

3. Controlling the density or spacing of visual stimuli.[187] In other words, change the distance between adjacent stimuli.

4. Providing consistent feedback to the patient about his performance of visual scanning tasks. The patient is progressed by gradually decreasing any of these cues.

---

* Reproduced with permission from Santa Clara Valley Medical Center, San Jose, California.

Specific Training Activities

1. Assuming that improvement in one task will carry over into another (i.e., function), have the patient perform tasks such as the following:
a. Cross out target letters (e.g., all A's) in the paragraph of a magazine, newspaper article, or scanning worksheet designed by the therapist. Utilize the retraining principles of anchoring, pacing, density, and feedback.
b. Complete paper mazes, puzzles, or other activities that require scanning ability.
2. Applying a functional approach:
a. Have the patient scan his room or clinic for specified items.
b. Take the patient to a community setting, such as a grocery, department, drug, or hardware store. In a particular section of the store, have the patient locate and retrieve a set of items as listed by the therapist.
c. Locate names, items, and prices, as specified by the therapist, in the classified ads of the newspaper.
d. Locate names, numbers, or addresses in a local telephone directory.
3. Some clinicians advocate the use of computers as an effective treatment tool for visual scanning retraining.

Saccadic Eye Movements

Saccadic eye movements are sequenced rapid eye movements. Saccades refer to the ability to localize stimuli and involve peripheral vision. By consciously "turning off" one's peripheral vision, saccadic eye movements become more efficient and organized. Saccadic eye movements are used extensively in reading.

Lesion site: area 8 of the frontal cortex.[74]

Evaluation of Saccadic Eye Movements

TEST NO. 1: King-Devick Test[149]
Description: This test consists of one demonstration card and three test cards. (See Figures 2-2 through 2-4.*) Subtest I consists of randomly spaced numbers connected by horizontal lines; Subtests II and III do not include any lines.

The patient is asked to call out the numbers in order as fast as possible, following the arrows.

Scoring: The time for completion is recorded in whole seconds, and the number of errors is noted for each subtest.

This test has established norms (sample=1202) for ages 6 to 14.[149]

To improve validity, rule out impaired visual attention and aphasia as causes of poor performance.

---

* Reproduced with permission from the Bernell Corp., P.O. Box 4637, South Bend, Indiana 46634.

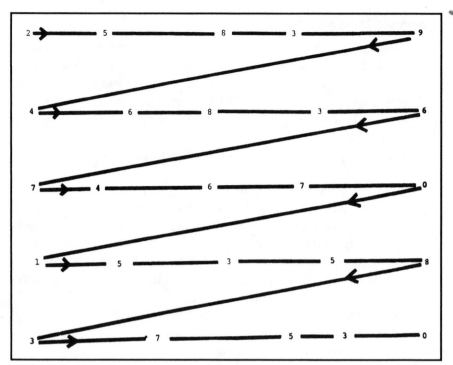
Figure 2-2. King-Devick Demonstration Card.

Figure 2-3. King-Devick Test I.

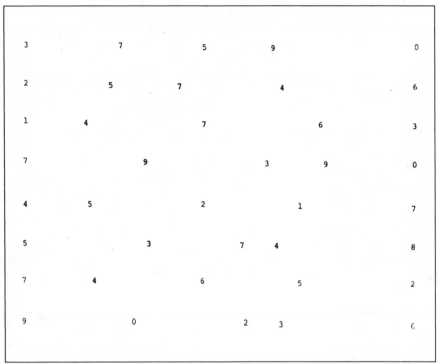

Figure 2-4. King-Devick Test II.

Treatment of Deficits in Saccadic Eye Movements

1. Believing that improvement in one task will transfer into another, have the patient perform such activities as calling out or pointing to letters from two columns printed on either side of a page (Figure 2-5). To progress with the activity, the column of printed letters should be printed closer to the center of the page (Figure 2-6). This activity can be adapted further by placing the columns on a blackboard and changing the distance between the columns as the patient progresses.[249]

2. In an attempt to utilize sensory input combined with a motor output, utilize vestibular based movement activities in conjunction with demands for saccadic skills. For instance, have the patient roll one-quarter turn and identify a number or letter that has been randomly placed on a suspended ball.[249] Repeat the activity with a half turn, a three-quarter turn, and so on.

3. Some clinicians advocate the use of videogames and computers for the remediation of basic oculomotor deficits.

4. Utilizing a multimodality approach, apply several of the treatment strategies described.

Figure 2-5. Saccadic Eye Movement Worksheet 1

1 F	T 1
2 N	U 2
3 P	P 3
4 V	X 4
5 R	A 5
6 M	W 6
7 H	F 7
8 O	B 8
9 S	Z 9
10 T	L 10
11 K	E 11

Figure 2-6. Saccadic Eye Movement Worksheet 2

1 X	C 1
2 M	T 2
3 A	W 3
4 F	B 4
5 O	L 5
6 Z	H 6
7 P	N 7
8 W	S 8
9 C	X 9
10 G	R 10
11 N	V 11

Visual Fields

The normal monocular field of vision is approximately 60 degrees upward, 60 degrees inward, 70 to 75 degrees downward, and 100 to 110 degrees outward.[116] This field of vision can be altered following a stroke. The type of deficit the patient sustains depends on the location and size of the lesion. Visual field deficits may be seen in patients with or without associated visual neglect.

Lesion site: The types of common visual field deficits and associated lesion sites are illustrated in Figure 2-7.[60]

Evaluation of Visual Fields

TEST NO. 1: Confrontation Testing—Without Eye Patch*[,247]

Both eyes together: The therapist sits directly in front of the patient, about 18 inches away. The patient fixates on the examiner's nose. If possible, the patient's back

---

* Reproduced with permission from Santa Clara Valley Medical Center, San Jose, California.

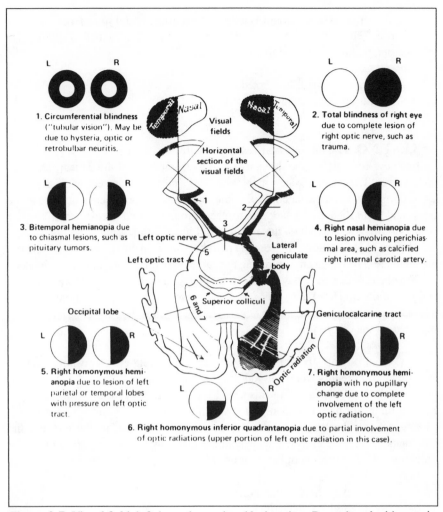

Figure 2-7. Visual field deficits and associated lesion sites. Reproduced with permission.

should be to the light with the patient facing a dark uniform background behind the examiner. The test objects are two dull black 2-foot wands with white balls on the end. When testing with both wands together, the therapist is checking for the extinction phenomenon. The therapist alternates using one or two wands and moves either or both in from the right or left periphery, at times simultaneously, in the simulated arc of the visual fields, meeting in the center, toward fixation. The patient is asked to indicate whether he sees one target or two while he focuses on the examiner's nose. He is also asked where they are located. The therapist should alternate the pattern by presenting one target in the right field, one in the left, and then both together. Repeat a total of nine times. The target should be moved again in the three planes: eye level, forehead, and below chin level (three times each level).

Directions:

1. (Verbal Patient) "I want you to keep both eyes on my nose. Tell me if you can see one ball or two and where it is located. You can point to where it is if you wish. Do you see one ball or two? Where?"

2. (Nonverbal Patient) "Before I tell you what to do, I want you to keep both eyes on my nose. Tell me if you see one ball or two by pointing to the one(s) you see. Do you see one ball or two? Point to what you see."

Scale:

1—Present, visual field loss noted.

0—Absent, no visual field loss noted.

TEST NO. 2: Confrontation Testing—With Eye Patch.[*,247]

Each eye separately: The therapist sits directly in front of the patient, about 18 inches away. The patient fixates on the examiner's nose with one eye while the other eye is covered with an eye patch. If possible, the patient's back should again be to the light, and there should be a dark uniform background behind the examiner. The test object used is a white ball on the end of a dull black 2-foot wand.

The test object is moved in from the periphery of the patient's field (from the left and then the right) in an arc simulating the curve of an imaginery sphere (perimeter).

The object is moved slowly in at eye level first, and then repeated at forehead level and just below chin level (nine times). The patient is asked to respond verbally or with a gesture as soon as he can see the target. The eye patch is then switched and the test repeated on the other eye.

Directions:

1. (Verbal Patient) "For this test I want you to keep your eye on my nose. Say yes as soon as you see this white ball move in from the side."

2. (Nonverbal Patient) "For this test, I want you to keep your eye on my nose. Raise a finger (or hand) as soon as you see the white ball move in from the side."

Observe whether there is sufficient visual attentiveness for this test and the quadrants of each eye in which the patient has difficulty in attending to stimuli. The problem can be central, peripheral, or anywhere in the field.

Scale:

1—Present, visual field deficit noted.

0—Absent, all visual fields intact.

Reliability: Both the described confrontation tests, when given alone (i.e., not in conjunction with additional gross visual skills testing), did not reach an acceptable level (i.e., $r > 0.75$) of inter-rater reliability in a study conducted on a sample of patients who had sustained head trauma.[23] These tests, however, utilized as part of an overall gross visual skills evaluation, did have good inter-rater reliability ($r = 0.82$ for overall gross visual skills evaluation). In addition, interitem correlations between the two tests revealed an almost perfect correlation ($r = 0.97$). This almost perfect correlation suggests that administering both tests (i.e., with and without the patch) provides no additional information. Further research should indicate whether deleting one of these tests is justified in order to shorten the evaluation.

Confrontation testing, similar to the tests described, is commonly utilized as a measure of visual fields in the adult patient with head trauma.[9,21,116,224,228]

To improve validity, rule out aphasia, poor visual attention, and scanning as causes of poor performance.

---

* Reproduced with permission from Santa Clara Valley Medical Center, San Jose, California.

Treatment for Visual Field Deficits

1. Applying the concept that environment can affect performance;
   a. Place a bedside table, comb, newspaper, and any commonly used objects on the side of poor vision, forcing the patient to look to that side.
   b. Or, if the patient is unable to compensate for his visual field deficit, to increase functional independence, place all necessary items within the patient's field of vision.
2. Utilizing a multimodality approach, provide verbal, auditory (e.g., bell, finger snapping) and tactile cuing to encourage the patient to look to the affected side.
3. Activities as described in the treatment of visual scanning and unilateral neglect deficits are also helpful in training the patient to compensate for a visual field deficit.
4. Some researchers believe that visual retraining involving light sensitivity measures and measures of saccadic localization in deficit fields can actually increase visual function.[246] These researchers' findings, however, were not replicated in similar studies.[17]

Visual Neglect

In addition to or in the absence of a visual field deficit, the stroke patient may exhibit visual neglect. Visual neglect may be seen in conjunction with spatial neglect or body neglect. The patient may ignore one of two objects held in intact visual fields on either side of the midline when presented simultaneously.[173] Neglect may occur not only for midline opposite stimuli, but for contralateral upper and lower quadrants as well.[123] For example, a lower left quadrant stimulus can cause a simultaneous stimulus in the upper right quadrant to be neglected.[123]

Lesion site: Visual neglect deficits have been associated with frontal lobe damage[123] and left or right occipitoparietal and parietal damage.[69,190]

Evaluation of Visual Neglect

TEST NO. 1: Alternating Simultaneous Stimuli*,[247]
Procedure: The therapist is seated at arm's length directly facing the patient. The patient is instructed to focus on the therapist's nose. Using the index fingers of both

---

* Reproduced with permission from Santa Clara Valley Medical Center, San Jose, California.

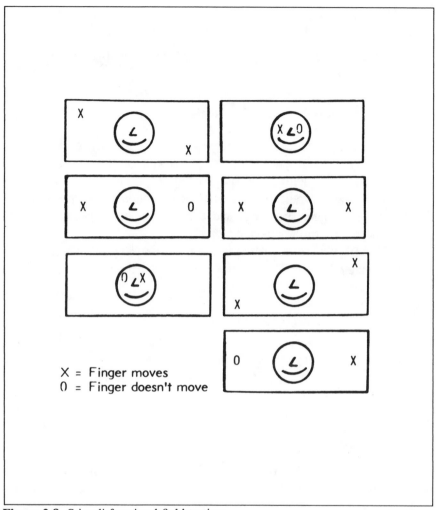

Figure 2-8. Stimuli for visual field testing.

hands approximately 8 inches in front of the patient's face, as in Figure 2-8, the therapist wiggles one or two fingers two times, a total of seven to 10 trials:

X = Finger moves.

o = Finger does not move.

Ask the patient to indicate which finger he sees moving, by either pointing or a verbal response.

Note: The rating should not overlap with the patient's field cut, as you would be sketching field loss and not neglect. Test for neglect within the patient's visual field and on the border of the field deficit if present.

Directions: "For this test, keep your eyes on my nose at all times. Tell me how many fingers I move—one or two. Point to what moved."

Observe whether the patient is able to attend consistently to visual stimuli presented simultaneously or whether he neglects right or left stimuli. Note: Visual confrontation on only the affected side may reveal no apparent neglect. However, subsequent simultaneous confrontation may show visual neglect of stimuli in the presence of intact peripheral vision.

Scale:

1—Present, visual spatial neglect noted.

0—Absent, attends to visual stimuli correctly.

TEST NO. 2: Line Bisection Test*.[247]

Procedure: Using the two line bisection worksheets placed and taped end to end directly in front of the patient with the taped section at midline on the table, ask the patient to draw a short line through the middle of each one of the lines (use a pen). Choose a line in the middle of the page to demonstrate. Do not give clues regarding whether the patient has marked all of them, and do not allow movement of the paper. Save the sheet, and mark where the top of the page is.

Time: 90 seconds for the whole task (use as a guideline).

Directions: "Draw a short line through the middle of each one of the lines that you see. Watch me; this is what I want you to do. Begin." (Do not give clues.)

Observe whether the patient's lines are constantly off midline or whether he draws all the lines on one side of the paper first, and whether he completely misses one area of the page. Poor performance may indicate hemianopsia, visual neglect, poor visual scanning, or all these problems.

Scale:

2—Severely impaired, any mark over ½ inch off midline, any missed line, greater than 90 seconds.

1—Minimally impaired, any mark over ¼ inch off midline, greater than 90 seconds.

0—Intact, all marks within ¼ inch of the midline, within 90 seconds.

To improve validity; rule out aphasia, decreased visual attention, and scanning and visual field deficit as causes of poor performance.

Reliability: Tests similar to the ones described have traditionally been used as tests of visual neglect.[224,228]

The line bisection test, when given as an isolated test, did not reach an acceptable level ($r < 0.75$) of inter-rater reliability in a study conducted on a sample of head trauma patients.[23] This test, however, utilized as part of an overall gross visual skills evaluation, did have good inter-rater reliability ($r = 0.82$ for overall gross visual skills evaluation).

Treatment of Visual Neglect

1. Utilizing a multimodality approach, provide verbal, auditory, and tactile cuing to decrease neglect and increase the patient's awareness of the deficit.

2. Activities as described in the treatment of visual scanning and unilateral neglect are also helpful in visual neglect training.

---

* Reproduced with permission from Santa Clara Valley Medical Center, San Jose, California.

CHAPTER III

The Apraxias

Apraxia is the inability to perform certain skilled purposeful movements in the absence of loss of motor power, sensation, or coordination. Seldom is the term *apraxia* used without a clarifying descriptor. A common occurrence following cerebral vascular accidents, apraxia results from cerebral lesions of either or both hemispheres and may take several forms, including constructional, motor, ideomotor, ideational, verbal (also see under *Aphasia* (Chapter VII), and dressing. Two or more types of apraxias usually occur together; only rarely is one type found in isolation.[125]

Constructional Apraxia

Constructional apraxia is the impairment in producing designs in two or three dimensions, by copying, drawing, or constructing, whether upon command or spontaneously. Constructional apraxia results from lesions in either cerebral hemisphere and limits the patient's ability to perform purposeful acts while using objects in his environment.[128]

A controversy exists about the occurrence of constructional apraxia among patients with right- and left-sided brain damage. It is widely believed that patients with right-sided damage show a greater incidence of the deficit.[189] However, others hypothesize an equal distribution of the symptoms of both right and left groups.[79] The authors, hypothesizing an equal distribution of symptoms in both groups, insist that aphasic patients often have the deficit but are not included in test groups for patients with left-sided brain damage, since they are frequently either confused or unable to understand directions.

Although patients with both right and left hemiplegia display this deficit, a distinct difference between the two groups (supported more by observation of quality of response than by objective perceptual testing[79]) has been widely described in the literature. It seems the apractic patients with right-sided lesions, with or without visual field deficits, are characterized by a visual-spatial disability, such that they lack perspective, the exact location of a figure in space, and the ability to analyze parts in relation to each other.[79,101,121,189] Apractic patients with left-sided lesions have spatial problems only if a visual field deficit exists simultaneously, but overall exhibit an executive or planning problem.[79,101,121,189] Thus, these patients, regardless of whether they are able to see things in correct perspective, have trouble in initiating a planned sequence of movements when trying to construct an object.

Patients with right-sided cerebral damage tend to be less hesitant in their drawings and use a piecemeal approach rather than an orderly one.[101] They frequently draw on the diagonal, neglect the left side of the drawing, and have no particular way for using the space on the page.[189] Their designs are often very complex, often unrecognizable, but do include many pieces of the drawing scattered without proper spatial relationships to one another.[167,189] Frequently, lines in the drawing are overscored in an attempt to correct or finish the task.[101] Their drawings show that they have a great deal of difficulty with perspective, and constructing anything with three dimensions, such as blocks or bricks, is extremely difficult.[122] These patients are usually not helped by the presence of a model and when given some landmarks, e.g., part of the drawing filled in, their work is unaffected or they are made more confused.[121,189] Short-term visual memory is hypothesized to be poor and the patient seems unable to keep the model in mind.[53,229] After several trials at a particular task, no learning appears to take place.[121]

On the other hand, patients with left-sided damage tend to be very hesitant in their task and produce designs of great simplicity.[167] They often cannot draw angles, their designs are poor in outline, and they have apparent difficulty in execution.[101] These patients seem to have more general intellectual impairment, and it is thought that their ability to establish the program task is lost or diminished.[89,121] However, their performance is often facilitated by the presence of a model, and often they tend to move closer and closer to it (called the closing-in effect by Mayer-Gross[163]) until finally their copy is superimposed on the model.[189] Landmarks, i.e., part of the picture filled in, appear helpful.[121] After several trials, these patients seem to learn the task and can repeat it more easily.[121] Memories for visual and auditory images are thought to be short,[53,229] and thus drawing to command or from memory is affected more than copying a model.

Functionally, constructional apraxia has been related to body scheme problems and often results in dressing difficulties and difficulties in daily living skills.[24,150,186,238] Lorenze and Cancro,[150] using the WAIS block design and object assembly subtests, found that patients who did poorly on these tests did not acquire dressing and grooming skills even after practice in dressing. In patients with right-sided lesions, the presence of severe constructional apraxia with perceptual problems has been found to relate to the same lack of independence in daily living skills.[112]

Constructional apraxia for the nondominant hemisphere may also be a syndrome that occurs in apractognosia.

Lesion site: occipitoparietal lobe of either hemisphere.[165]

Evaluation for Constructional Apraxia

TEST NO. 1: Copying Designs—Two Dimensional
Description: The therapist hands the patient paper and pencil and asks him to copy the design on the stimulus card. A separate sheet of paper is used to copy each stimulus card. There are several variations on this test, none of them standardized. For example:

1. Copy a previously drawn line drawing of a house (Figure 3-1), a flower, and a clock face.[112]

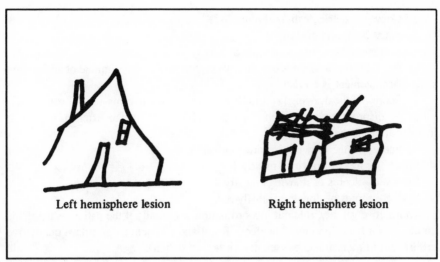

Figure 3-1. Example of imparied performance in drawing a house.

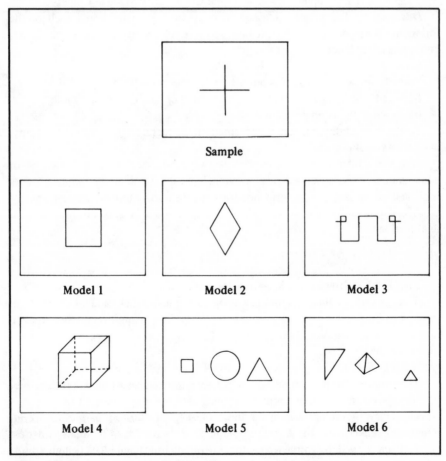

Figure 3-2. Copy geometric designs test.[150]

2. Copy geometric designs (Figure 3-2).

Scoring: Nonstandardized.

Each drawing is scored on a scale of 1 to 3.

1. Score 1 if the drawing is essentially correct, no lines are omitted or added, and spatial arrangement is correct.

2. Score 2 if the drawing is partially defective owing to omissions of some lines, rotations, disproportions between single parts, but not to such an extent as to prevent identification of the figure.

3. Score 3 if the drawing is unrecognizable.

Intact—scores of drawings mostly 1.

Impaired—scores of drawings mostly 2.

Severe—scores of drawings mostly 3.

To improve validity, rule out incoordination, especially if the patient is using his nondominant hand (unilateral neglect). Right and left hemiplegics have qualitative differences in their drawings (see description of deficit).

TEST NO. 2: Graphic Designs—Santa Clara Valley Medical Center[247]

Description: The patient is asked to copy from prepared cards each of the following: horizontal line, vertical line, cross, circle, square, triangle, diamond, cube, house, and clock.

Scoring:

Severely impaired—design is almost totally unrecognizable.

Impaired—design lacks perspective, is rotated or partly unrecognizable.

Intact—design is copied accurately.

To improve validity, rule out incoordination, unilateral neglect, visual field cuts, and other visual problems.

Reliability: Inter-rater reliability ($r = 0.98$) was established for this test in a study of adult patients who sustained head trauma.[23] In the same study frequency data indicated no variance in performance for copying horizontal and vertical lines, a cross, a square, and a triangle. All other items appeared to be good discriminators of dysfunction.

TEST NO. 3: Matchstick Designs[112]

Description: The therapist makes a design using matchsticks and asks the patient to copy it. The designs should vary in complexity, from using two wooden kitchen matches to nine matches. There is no standardized form of this test. The therapist makes up the designs.

Scoring: Subjective.

Intact—patient copies all designs correctly within a reasonable length of time.

To improve validity, rule out unilateral neglect, motor apraxias.

Reliability: A refined matchstick design test[247] was utilized as part of a constructional praxis subtest in a study of adult patients with head trauma.[23] Intertest correlations showed the correlation between the matchstick and block design tests to be extremely high ($r = 0.92$). This high correlation ($r = 0.9222$) had also been found in a study conducted by Baum and Hall.[24] This combined research indicates that administering both a matchstick design and a block design test is unnecessary duplication. In addition, item analysis revealed a higher overall reliability when the matchstick design test was deleted rather than the block design test. It is therefore recommended that a matchstick design test be utilized only if a block design test is unavailable.

TEST NO. 4: Block Bridges[252]
Description: Using 1-inch cube blocks, the therapist builds a three-block bridge in front of the patient and then asks him to copy it. If the patient does it correctly, the therapist builds a five-block bridge and has the patient copy it and then a seven-block bridge and lets the patient copy it.
Scoring: Subjective.
Intact—bridges are correct.
To improve validity, rule out motor apraxias and incoordination.

TEST NO. 5: Block Designs, Santa Clara Valley Medical Center[247]
Description: The patient is asked to duplicate block designs from prepared models.
Scoring:
Severely impaired—design is almost totally unrecognizable.
Impaired—design is rotated, wrong number of blocks, or partly recognizable.
Intact—design is copied accurately.
To improve validity, rule out motor apraxias.
Reliability: Inter-rater reliability (r = 0.96) was established for this test in a study of adult head trauma patients.[23] In addition, item analysis indicated a high degree of test reliability (alpha = 0.87) for this test given in conjunction with the Santa Clara Valley Medical Center graphic design test.[23]

TEST NO. 6: Benton's Three-dimensional Constructional Praxis Test[28,186]
Description: The patient is asked to copy block constructions composed of blocks of various sizes (Figure 3-3). The test set of 29 blocks is organized in a shallow box (Figure 3-4) and placed on the patient's unaffected side. The sample is placed in front of the patient and he is told to copy it. The therapist demonstrates first and then returns the blocks to the box. The patient then tries to copy the model. If he is successful, the blocks are returned to the box and first test model is placed in front of him at a 45 degree angle. The blocks of all the models are glued together for easy handling. The patient is given five minutes to copy the model. Then the blocks are returned to the box and the procedure is repeated for the second test model.
Scoring: Nonstandardized.
Each block is scored one point if correct and zero points if incorrect according to whether it was:
Omitted—the block not included in the construction.

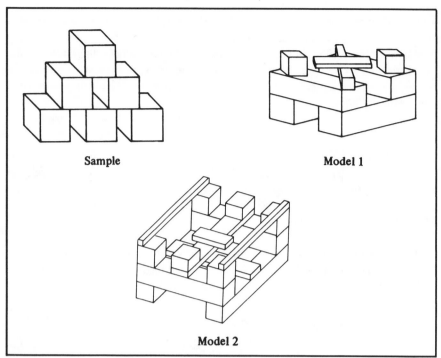

Sample

Model 1

Model 2

Figure 3-3. Benton's three dimensional constructional praxis test.[28]

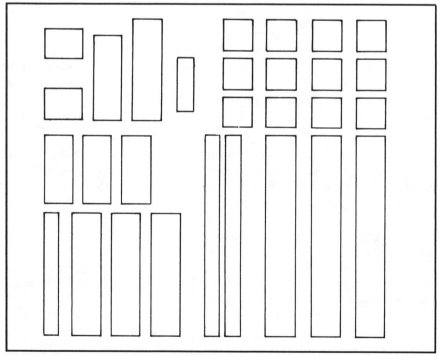

Figure 3-4. Arrangement of blocks for the three dimensional construction test.

42

Substituted—the patient substituted a block of a different size from the one in the model.

Displaced—the block placed on the wrong corner or section of the figure.

Blocks that were correctly placed but not exactly lined up with those immediately above or below them, e.g., slightly rotated, are considered correct. Scoring is done in layers, from the bottom layer up, and blocks are scored in relation to those below them. If one layer is omitted, the next layer is scored in relation to those below it.

Intact—score of 22-23 (90 percent of normal controls).

Impaired—score of 20-21 (9 percent of control group).

Severe—score of 19 or below (1 percent of control group).[9]

To improve validity, rule out motor apraxias.

TEST NO. 7: The Bender-Gestalt Test[183]

Description: The patient is given a blank piece of paper and a pencil. He is shown nine cards, one at a time, and asked to draw the design he sees on the card. He draws all nine designs on the one piece of paper.

Scoring: Standardized. In testing its reliability, the authors report a test-retest correlation of $r = 0.71$ and a score reliability of $r = 0.90$. This test has elaborate directions for scoring. To learn how to score it, one must consult the manual. However, one can make observations from the results even if it is not scored.

To improve validity, rule out unilateral neglect, hemianopsia, poor eyesight, poor coordination due to paresis, or use of nondominant hand.

Other Tests. Almost any constructional task can be used to evaluate this problem. Since none of them have been standardized in patients with strokes and some of them have been described elsewhere in this chapter, we will only list some of the more common ones here: copying pegboard designs, puzzles, copying block designs similar to designs on the Wechsler Adult Intelligence Scale, Draw-A-Man Test, Frostig's Spatial Relations Test.

Validity of Constructional Apraxia Tests. Benton[28] believes that the various "constructional apraxia" tests are not necessarily testing the same skill. He found that his Visual Retention Test (a test of copying geometric figures) correlated only weakly with his Three-Dimensional Praxis Test. Pehoski[186] also found only a weak correlation between her copy drawing test and Benton's Three-Dimensional Praxis Test.

The various tests vary in complexity, in the type of movement and dexterity required to do the task, in the demands of higher intellectual function, and in the involvement of two or three spatial dimensions. For example, the task of copying geometric designs requires more precise graphic movements and a higher degree of sensorimotor integration than block building or matchstick arranging.[28]

Treatment for Constructional Apraxia

1. Assuming that improvement on one task will transfer to similar tasks, have the patient practice simple copying or construction tasks.

For examples of copying tasks, see the treatment section under Spatial Relations Deficit.

2. For patients with lesions on the dominant side of the brain, see whether they are helped by the use of landmarks in very simple designs. Gradually reduce landmarks for simple designs and move on to more complicated ones. Move from two dimensional designs to three dimensional ones.[121]

For patients with nondominant side lesions, start with extremely simple designs, perhaps just an X or a T. Then move on to more complicated ones.

3. Provide additional proprioceptive and kinesthetic input by having the patient draw designs in a clayboard rather than with a paper and pencil.

Dressing Apraxia

Dressing apraxia is the inability to dress oneself because of a disorder in body scheme and/or spatial relations. This apraxia relates more to body scheme and spatial deficits than to a difficulty in the motor performance of dressing.[78] The patient makes mistakes of orientation in putting the clothes on backwards, upside-down, or inside out.[4] Often the patients with right-sided lesions will neglect to dress the left side of the body or put both legs in the same pant leg. The following is an excerpt from Charlene Pehoski's thesis describing a patient with dressing apraxia trying to put on a shirt.[186]

Case 1—Left Hemiplegic

(1) The subject was unable to find the correct sleeve. He looked at the shirt in a puzzled manner and finally put his involved arm into a sleeve, but it was the wrong sleeve. (2) He then had some difficulty getting the sleeve up the involved extremity, but he finally managed to slide it past the elbow and onto the involved shoulder. (3) He then reached around his back as a normal response to find the other sleeve. Since the correct sleeve had not been used at the beginning, the second arm hole was not in back as it should have been, but remained in front. He then came back to the material in front of him and found the second arm hole and put his uninvolved extremity in. The shirt was then on as if it were to be buttoned down the back. He looked puzzled for a moment and then put the material that was in front over his head to the back. Now he

had the bulk of the material behind his neck with the two shirt tails hanging over his shoulder in front. Feeling at the back of his neck, he asked, "Where is the collar?" After several seconds of fumbling for the collar and trying to pull the shirt down, he said, "I've fouled up somewhere along the line. The collar is nowhere." (Total time: three minutes, 34 seconds.)

Dressing apraxia may also be a syndrome that occurs in apractognosia.

Lesion site: occipital or parietal lobe, more often in the nondominant hemisphere.[165]

Evaluation for Dressing Apraxia

The test for this is strictly a functional one. Ask the patient to take off or put on a shirt and watch his performance. Does he have trouble in deciding where to begin or where to find the right armhole? Does he neglect to dress the left half of his body (indication of unilateral neglect)? Does he put the shirt on inside out or backwards? Does he button it so the buttons are not aligned correctly? All these are signs of dressing apraxia and not just the inability to dress because of motor paralysis. Because there is usually a high degree of correlation between dressing and constructional apraxia, some people have used tests of constructional apraxia to evaluate dressing apraxia.[150,238]

Treatment for Dressing Apraxia

Basically, the therapist teaches the patient a set pattern for dressing, trying to find a way that requires the least rotation of the garment and is most like the patient's habitual way of dressing. The therapist also teaches cognitive cues that help the patient distinguish right from left or front from back. The patient gets into a routine, practicing the same pattern day after day, until he learns it.[251,255]

Here are some cues to pass on to your patients:

1. If the patient has trouble positioning the garment, tell him to place his shirt down on the bed, buttons face down, or his pants on his lap, zipper face up. Initial positioning of the garment is especially important if patient confuses right and left.

2. Use labels to distinguish back from front and right from wrong side.

3. If garment does not have distinguishing labels, the therapist can color code the garment for right-left, back-front, and wrong side-right side.[255]

4. If patient has trouble matching buttons to the right buttonhole, tell him to start at the bottom of the shirt and find the last

button and match it to the last buttonhole. Continue matching upward from there. Or the therapist can color code the bottom button and buttonhole.[251]

5. Have patient circle the button with his finger to feel that he has it all the way through the buttonhole.[251]

Motor Apraxia

Motor apraxia is believed to be a loss of kinesthetic memory patterns that results in the patient's inability to perform a purposeful motor task on command, although it is apparent that the patient understands the concept and purpose of the task.[60] Motor apraxia appears to be a defect in execution.[60] This patient may be able to carry out simple motor tasks automatically, but cannot complete a complicated sequence. In observing the patient, motor apraxia and ideomotor apraxia may appear the same; however, lesion sites for the two generally are different.[60]

Lesion site: frontal lobe of either hemisphere, precentral gyrus.[60]

Ideomotor Apraxia

Ideomotor apraxia is the inability to imitate gestures or perform a purposeful motor task on command even though the patient fully understands the idea or concept of the task.[128] These patients, although unable to perform on command, retain kinesthetic memory patterns and the ability to carry out many old habitual motor tasks automatically.[17] However, they have a problem in motor planning with a loss of skilled sequence of movement and characteristically persevere in their movements.[60] For instance, if asked to write with a pencil, the patient could describe the act and recognize it, yet may not pick up the pencil and begin to write. However, at another time he might pick up the pencil and paper and start to write spontaneously.

Lesion site: parietal lobe of dominant hemisphere, supramarginal gyrus.[60,165]

Ideational Apraxia

Ideational apraxia is the inability to carry out activities automatically or on command because the patient no longer understands the concept of the act.[128] The mental process for conceptual sequencing that allows one to relate the symbolisms of object names and visual imagery to a related motor performance is lost.[78] Frequently complex acts cannot be performed whereas simple isolated acts or parts of acts remain. In responding to a command, the more hypothetical the request, the more difficulty the patient has.[78] He cannot pretend to perform an act or describe the function of an object. For example, if given a cigarette and a match and told to light the cigarette, the patient may put the match in his mouth or put the unlighted match to the cigarette. He also cannot describe the match's function.

Infrequently the ideational or conceptual objective of a motor performance is lost while the motor performance remains intact because the motor sequence belongs to the intact hemisphere, whereas the ideational sequence is found in the damaged hemisphere. Denny-Brown[78] refers to this syndrome as adextrous apraxia. For example, a left-handed man has learned to write with his right hand. After a right-sided brain lesion, he is unable to conceptualize and form an intelligible word; however, he retains the skill to form written letters with his right hand.[78]

Lesion site: parietal lobe of dominant hemisphere or diffuse brain damage as seen following arteriosclerosis.[60,165]

Evaluation of Motor, Ideomotor, and Ideational Apraxias

These apraxias are very similar and difficult to differentiate. The test is the same for them; only quality of the response varies slightly. When asked to do a task, a person with motor or ideomotor apraxia would not be able to do it on command, but could do it automatically at the appropriate time. A person with ideational apraxia could not do it even automatically, although he has the motor capacity to do it.

TEST NO. 1: Goodglass Test for Apraxia[109]

Description: This test consists of a series of tasks that the therapist asks the patient to do. If the patient fails on command, the therapist asks the patient to imitate her doing the tasks. If the patient still fails, and where applicable, the therapist asks the patient to do the task with real objects. The authors believe that this is the descending order of difficulty for apraxia patients. Often a patient uses his body parts as an object, e.g., his fist as a hammer, when asked to hammer a nail. He should be told to "pretend to hold the hammer." If he can correct this on verbal command, it is contraindicative of apraxia. The following is a list of tasks:

Buccal-facial
   1. Cough.
   2. Sniff.
   3. Blow out a match.
   4. Suck through a straw.
   5. Puff out your cheeks.
Limb
   1. Wave goodbye.
   2. Beckon "come here."
   3. Finger on lip for "shsh."
   4. Salute.

5. Signal "stop."
6. Brush teeth.
*7. Shave.
*8. Hammer.
*9. Saw board.
*10. Use screwdriver.

Whole body
1. How does a boxer stand?
2. How does a golfer stand?
3. How does a soldier march in place?
4. How do you shovel snow?
5. Stand up, turn around twice, and sit down.

Scoring: Subjective.

Intact—patient did most of the tasks correctly on verbal request without being given the actual object.

Impaired—patient did most of the tasks correctly only when given the actual object.

Severely impaired—patient could not do the tasks even when presented with the actual object.

To improve validity, rule out incomprehension of directions.

TEST NO. 2: Ayres' Imitation of Postures (subtest of Southern California Sensory Integration Tests)[14]

Description: The therapist and patient sit opposite each other in chairs without arms. The patient is asked to mirror image a series of 12 positions or postures demonstrated by the therapist. Nonmirror image responses are counted as correct, but the patient is told to give a mirror image thereafter.

Scoring: This test has been standardized for children aged 4.0 to 8.11 years. In testing for reliability, Ayres reports that the test-retest correlations range from $r = 0.29$ to 0.74. This test is scored subjectively for adults.

Intact—patient assumes all postures correctly in a reasonable length of time.

To improve validity, rule out paralysis or paresis of affected side, unilateral neglect, hemianopsia.

TEST NO. 3: The Solet Test for Apraxia[†,215]

Description: This is a 40-item evaluation technique is designed to further professional understanding of apraxia itself as well as for use in treatment planning. It identifies two variations of apraxia, ideational and ideomotor, by differenting the level of concreteness of impaired actions. Gestures, object use, demonstration of use of missing object, and nonrepresentational movements are included. Commands are

---

*When used with a female patient, say, "How would a man . . . ."

† The Solet Test for Apraxia is available through its author: Jo M. Solet, MOT, OTR, 5 Channing Road, Newton Center, Massachusetts 02159.

presented to distinguish three areas of possible body part involvement: buccal-facial, right or left (or both) upper extremities, and the whole body. The ability to follow verbal directions, to select described actions from a series of demonstrations, and to imitate the examiner are evaluated.

Scoring: Nonstandardized. The test supplies a structure for detailed examination of the actual individual client's apraxic response, rather than only indicating intact or impaired praxis. Response characteristics discussed include groping and hesitation, improvement on imitations, and displaced plane of movement. The test is followed by a series of treatment implications.

To improve validity, rule out incomprehension of the directions, paralysis or paresis of the affected side.

TEST NO. 4: Praxis Test—Santa Clara Valley Medical Center[247]

Description: This is a 10-item test, which is administered to command, involving both imitation and real objects (items 1 to 5 only). Items include buccal-facial, unilateral and bilateral limb, and total body tasks.

Scoring:

Severely impaired—action is almost unrecognizable.

Impaired—action is carried out imperfectly (e.g., directional problems, hesitation) or with some delay.

Intact—action is carried out immediately and correctly.

To improve validity, rule out paresis of affected side, incoordination, unilateral neglect, and incomprehension of directions.

Reliability: Inter-rater reliability (r = 0.99) was established for this test with a sample of adult patients with head trauma.[23]

In addition, interitem correlations indicated a high degree of correlation between several test items (refer to Appendix A). Additional research should indicate whether administering all test items is unnecessary duplication.

Treatment for Motor, Ideomotor, and Ideational Apraxias

1. Provide proprioceptive, tactile, and kinesthetic input prior to and during a task. For example, take the patient's leg through the required motion to propel his wheelchair.

2. Keep verbal commands to a minimum, and place activity on a subcortical level. For example, instead of the verbal command, "Lock your brakes," say to the patient, "There's something on your brakes."

3. Identify specifically the type of apraxia that is present, e.g., unilateral limb, total body. Are movements away from the body or toward the body affected? Use this information in your treatment approach. For instance, the patient with unilateral or bilateral limb apraxia will do better with gross motor, total body activities and will do worse if activities are broken down into segments. For

example, in coming to standing, giving directions and breaking down the activity into segments, such as scooting, pushing, and leaning, will only serve to confuse the patient. A simple command, such as, "Get up," puts the activity on a more automatic total body level.

4. Activities should be performed in as nearly normal an environment as possible. For example, dressing should be done in the morning at the bedside instead of in the clinic in the middle of the day. If possible, cooking activities should be done in the home, or at least with familiar utensils.

5. Have the patient close his eyes and visualize the required movements before attempting to carry them out.

6. Provide support to the patient when he becomes frustrated. Explain to him that you know that he is not being uncooperative and that certain movements are difficult for him. Provide some activities during therapy that will assure the patient success.

Verbal Apraxia

Verbal apraxia is the difficulty in forming and organizing intelligible words, although the musculature required to do so remains intact. This differs from dysarthria in which the muscles are affected and the speech is slurred. These patients may be able to use the tongue for automatic acts such as chewing and swallowing, but may not be able to stick it out when asked. This seems to be a motor planning problem.[78]

Recent research has indicated that verbal apraxia involves not only a motor deficit but language and perceptual difficulties as well.[137]

Lesion site: frontal lobe of the left hemisphere.[78]

Evaluation and Treatment for Verbal Apraxia

Evaluation and treatment for verbal apraxia are usually done by the speech pathologist. However, if there is no speech pathologist available, a simple screening test can be used. First, ask the patient to lick his lips. If he cannot do so on command, put some honey or peanut butter on his lips and observe whether he automatically licks it off. If he can lick his lips automatically but not on command, he is probably apraxic. If he cannot lick them at all, he is probably dysarthric. The buccal/facial part of the Goodglass Test for Apraxia contains other tasks to use in a test for verbal apraxia.

Because the problem occurs only when the patient consciously tries to use his muscles, some therapists feel that there is no real effective therapy.[223]

CHAPTER IV

Body Image and Body Scheme Disorders

Body image and body scheme disturbances occur commonly and are thought to result in an alteration of the way a person understands himself, i.e., his illness, his body, or its parts.[128]

The terms body image and body scheme are often mistakenly used interchangeably in the literature and by therapists. However, an essential difference between the two terms exists, and it is important for the reader to understand this distinction.

Body image is the visual and mental memory image of one's body. It is the mental representation of one's body that expresses feelings and thoughts rather than representing an exact picture of the physical structure.[125]

The body scheme regulates the position of different muscles and parts of the body to each other at any given moment in time. Body scheme, on the other hand, is a postural model one has of oneself, having to do with how one perceives the position of the body and the relationship of body parts.[125] Body scheme is believed to be the basis for all motions, for one needs to know the parts of the body and their relationships in order to know what, where, and how to move oneself.[12]

Included in body image and body scheme disturbances are somatognosia, anosognosia-anosodiaphoria, unilateral neglect, right-left discrimination, and finger agnosia.

Somatognosia

Somatognosia, a disturbance in body scheme, is the lack of awareness of body structure and the failure to recognize one's parts and their relationship to each other. A patient who has such a deficit also has difficulties in his reference point to the outside world. A patient with this difficulty may have trouble using his contralateral limbs, may confuse the sides of the body, and may not differentiate properly his own body parts and those of the examiner.[211]

Macro- and microsomatognosia are disorders in body scheme that distort a person's perception of his own body. A patient may see his whole body or part of it as abnormally small (micro) or exceptionally large (macro). This may occur as a result of right or left hemisphere lesions.[139]

In patients who have somatognosia without an accompanying problem in spatial relations, the prospects for successfully attaining skills of daily living are high.[50]

Lesion site: usually the parietal lobe of the dominant hemisphere.[51]

Evaluation of Somatognosia

TEST NO. 1: Point to Body Parts on Command[39,156,165,247,250,251]
Description: Therapist asks patient to point or indicate in some way the body part

named on himself, on the examiner, and on a human figure, puzzle, or doll. There is no standardized form for this test. The therapist can make up the commands. Here are some examples excluding "left" and "right" from the command.

1. Show me your knees.
2. Show me your mouth.
3. Show me your stomach.
4. Show me your nose.
5. Show me your feet.
6. Show me your shoulders.
7. Show me your elbows.
8. Show me your hair.
9. Show me your back.

Scoring: Nonstandardized.

Intact—patient correctly indicates all parts named in a reasonable length of time.

Validity: Sauguet,[203] Boone,[39] Macdonald,[156] and Brown[47] use variations of this test to measure body scheme. It is used mainly to test a patient's verbal understanding. Sauguet separated his sample into left hemiplegics, right hemiplegics without receptive aphasia, and right hemiplegics with receptive aphasia. Only the patients with receptive aphasia made errors on this test. Boone found that if the words "right" and "left" were excluded from the command, most of the errors were eliminated.

Research conducted with adult patients sustaining head trauma on a variation of this test established inter-rater reliability ($r=0.94$).[23] Item analysis of this subtest given with four additional subtests (i.e., Draw-A-Person, Right/Left Discrimination, Body Puzzle, and Face Puzzle) indicated good internal consistency (coefficient alpha$=0.60$).*,[23]

To improve validity, rule out aphasia as a cause of poor performance.

TEST NO. 2: Point to Body Parts—Imitation[161,203]

Description: The patient is told to imitate movements of the examiner, who touches different parts of his own body. Mirror image responses are acceptable. There is no standardized form of this test. Therapists can make up their own commands. Touching six to 10 body parts is sufficient. For example.

1. Touch your left hand.
2. Touch your right cheek.
3. Touch your left leg.
4. Touch your left elbow.
5. Touch your right palm.
6. Touch your right knee.
7. Touch your left shoulder.
8. Touch your right ear.
9. Touch your right forearm.
10. Touch your left wrist.

---

* A coefficient alpha measure of 0.50 was considered acceptable for the establishment of reliability.

Scoring: Nonstandardized.

Intact—patient correctly indicates all parts named within a reasonable length of time.

Validity: This test eliminates most of the verbal problems of the last test. Indeed, in Sauguet's[203] study, 90 percent of the right hemiplegics with aphasia had a normal performance as compared with 100 percent of the right hemiplegics without aphasia and left hemiplegics.

To improve validity, rule out apraxia as a cause of poor performance.

TEST NO. 3a: Body Visualization and Space Concepts (Norm descriptive statistics available in adaptation by Taylor)[222].*

Description: The examiner reads questions to the patient. Instruct the patient to "Think of yourself sitting as you are now when answering the following questions."

1. Ordinarily, are a person's teeth inside or outside his mouth?
2. Are your legs below your stomach?
3. Which is farther from your nose—your feet or your stomach?
4. Is your mouth above your eyes?
5. Which is closer to your mouth—your neck or shoulder?
6. Is your shoulder between your neck and your elbow?
7. Are your fingers between your elbow and your hand?
8. Which is farther from your toes—your heel or elbow?
9. Which is nearer to your head—your arms or your legs?
10. Which is on top of your head—your hair or eyes?
11. Is your back behind you or in front of you?
12. Is your stomach behind you or in front of you?
13. Is your elbow above or below your shoulder?
14. Is your nose above or below your neck?

Scoring: Although this test has not been standardized for adults, Taylor[221] in the article, "Analysis of Dysfunction in the Left Hemiplegia Following Stroke," provides the following data. However, until a more extensive normative study can be done, interpretation of scores is nonstandardized.

Age	Number of Subjects	Mean Score*	Standard Deviation
50-64	90	27.5	1.3
65-74	60	26.9	1.2

*Scores combine accuracy and time.

---

* Developed by A.J. Ayres, ADI Auxiliary Publication Project, Document 8179, Library of Congress, Washington, D.C.

Intact—patient correctly answers all questions within a reasonable length of time. To improve validity, rule out aphasia as a cause of poor performance.

TEST NO. 3b: Body Revisualization

Macdonald[156] has devised a shorter version of this test in which the patient only has to answer "true" or "false." An expressive aphasia patient can indicate "true" or "false" by pointing to one of two cards marked "true" and "false."

Description: Ask the patient whether these statements are true or false:
1. Your mouth is below your chin.
2. Your eyes are above your forehead.
3. Your knees are below your hips.
4. Your hands are at the end of your arms.
5. You have one chin, one nose, and one mouth.

Scoring: Nonstandardized.

Intact—all correct within a reasonable length of time.

To improve validity, rule out receptive aphasia.

TEST NO. 4: Draw-A-Man[112,156,250,251]

Description: Patient is given a blank piece of paper and a pencil and is asked to draw a man.

Scoring: Nonstandardized.

The following scoring system is taken from Macdonald.[156] The Goodenough-Harris Drawing Test[108] and the Denver Developmental Screening Test[95] both have standardized scoring systems for children. The first is more complicated than Macdonald's; the second is less complicated. The second scoring system included in this section is from Zoltan et al.[247]

Scoring system no. 1: Total of four points for presence of all body parts.

Point distribution:

One point—head

One point—trunk

Two points—two arms if full figure, one arm if profile

Two points—two legs if full figure, one leg if profile

2. Total of three points for correct proportion of body parts to trunk.

Point distribution:

One point—area of head not more than one-half or less than one-half the length of the trunk

One point—at least one arm not longer than twice the length of the trunk or less than one-half the length of the trunk

One point—at least one leg not longer than twice the length of the trunk or less than the length of the trunk

3. Total of one point for correct postural alignment, i.e., figure in normal standing or sitting position.

4. Total of two points for correct juxtaposition of extremities with trunk.

Point distribution:

One point—arms emerge from upper one-half of trunk
One point—legs emerge from lower one-half of trunk
Intact—total score of 10 points
Scoring system no. 2:
Total of 10 body parts

Head	Right hand
Trunk	Left hand
Right arm	Right foot
Left arm	Left foot
Right leg	Left leg

Intact—scores 10
Minimally impaired—scores 6 to 9
Severely impaired—scores 5 or below

Reliability: Research conducted on a sample of patients with head trauma utilizing this scoring system established inter-rater reliability (r=0.86).[23] As noted with the pointing to body parts test, the Draw-A-Person Test, when given to adult patients with head trauma with four other subtests, had an overall reliability of coefficient alpha=0.60.[23]

To improve validity: This test is also used as a means of identifying or diagnosing unilateral neglect and anosognosia. It is a constructional task and therefore overlaps into disorders of spatial judgment and apraxia, which should be ruled out. The validity of this test as a test of body image is controversial. Maloney and Payne[161] treated a group of retarded teenagers with sensory-motor training based on the work of Kephart and pre- and post-tested them with three tests of body image including the Draw-A-Man Test. On the post-testing the group made significant gains on the two other tests of body image but not on the Draw-A-Man Test. They concluded that the test does not reflect changes in body image occurring as a result of sensory-motor training. The Draw-A-Man Test is also used as a personality projective test, i.e., to determine how one feels about one's body. Gregory and Aitken[112] found that depressed patients often drew a miserable looking man whose size was very small on the page. This test is also used as a test of intelligence.[108]

TEST NO. 5: Human Figure or Face Puzzle[112,156,247,251] (Figure 4-1)
Equipment: Pieces of felt or cardboard or Plexiglas cut out to represent (a) head, trunk, arms, legs; (b) hands and feet; and (c) large piece of black felt for background.
Description: The patient is asked to put together pieces to resemble a human figure after individual parts have first been identified for the patient. For example, "Here are the man's arms, legs, head, and trunk. See whether you can put him together." In a variation of this test, the patient is not told that it is a man but simply told to put the puzzle together.
Scoring: Subjective, nonstandardized.[247]
Intact—able to assemble puzzle in 1.5 minutes with no errors
Impaired—able to put four to 10 pieces together but takes more than 1.5 minutes
Severely impaired—able to put one to three pieces together correctly
Reliability: Research conducted on a sample of patients with head trauma utilizing

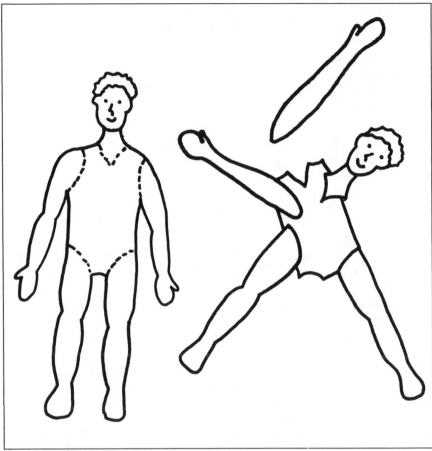

Figure 4-1. Left, human figure puzzle. Right, example of a severely impaired performance.

this scoring system established inter-rater reliability (r=0.84).[23] As noted with the previous body scheme tests, when given with the four other subtests, the overall reliability was good (alpha=0.60).[23]

To improve validity, rule out spatial-constructional disorders and figure-ground problems as causes of poor performance. This test is also used to test unilateral neglect and anosognosia.

TEST NO. 6: Face Puzzle[228]

Description: The patient is asked to put together pieces to resemble a human face.

Scoring: Nonstandardized.

To improve validity, rule out constructional disorders and figure-ground problems as causes of poor performance.

Reliability: Research conducted on a sample of patients with head trauma indicated no variation in subject performance and a high correlation with constructional praxis.[23]

Future research should indicate whether this is a meaningful test of body scheme.

58

Treatment for Somatognosia

1. In an attempt to associate sensory input with adaptive motor response, practice connecting specific stimulation with specific motor responses. For example:
   a. Using either his hand or a rough cloth the patient rubs a body part as it is named.[3,251]
   b. The patient imitates the body movements of therapist, e.g., right hand on left ear, left hand on right knee.[3]

2. Assuming that improvement in one task will transfer to similar tasks, practice particular tasks that reinforce body parts and their relation to one another. For example:
   a. The patient identifies body parts as they are touched by the therapist.[3]
   b. Quiz patient on body parts; e.g., show me or touch your knees.[250,251]
   c. Patient practices putting together a human figure puzzle.[251]

3. Utilizing a neurodevelopmental treatment approach:
   a. Incorporate into treatment bilateral activities that facilitate normal movement and improved body scheme.
   b. Provide appropriate handling techniques to educate the patient about what it feels like to move normally.

Unilateral Neglect

Unilateral neglect is the inability to integrate and use perceptions from the left side of the body or the left side of the environment. This deficit may occur independently of visual deficits or be compounded by left hemianopsia. However, it has been found that even in patients with seemingly intact visual fields, there is a reduction in flicker frequency, dark adaptation, and motion perception,[89] so that even patients with seemingly intact vision may, in fact, have a defect. A patient with unilateral neglect will ignore the left half of his body. For instance, he may forget to shave the left side of his face or dress his left side. Unilateral neglect may occur in the left half of his extrapersonal space so that the patient will neglect the food on the left side of the plate or read starting in the middle of the line. He may bump into things on his left or constantly be turning to his right.

Someone with unilateral neglect differs physically from a patient with a left homonymous hemianopsia because the former has seemingly intact fields of vision, whereas the latter has a blindness in the left-sided fields of both eyes. It appears that the patient with hemanopsia might still receive full or adequate sensation from his left side and may automatically compensate for his visual deficits.[125] On the other hand, the patient with unilateral neglect may have diminished sensation on his affected side, thus compounding the problem and "forgetting" that side. This patient is usually very slow in learning to compensate for his disability and, in fact, may never fully incorporate his left-sided personal and extrapersonal environment in his functioning.[125]

Unilateral neglect may also be a syndrome that occurs in apractognosia, a deficit consisting of several different apraxia and agnostic syndromes, all centering mainly around a lack of perspective.[122]

Lesion site: inferior parietal lobe of the right, nondominant hemisphere.[165]

Evaluation for Unilateral Neglect

TEST NO. 1a: Draw-A-Man, Draw-A-Clock[112]
Description: Patient is given separate sheets of blank paper for each task and told to "draw a man" and "draw a clock" in turn.
Scoring: Subjective.
Intact—drawings include all parts in proper place.
Impaired—some parts are missing from the left side, or body parts are thinner on left side, or parts are skewed to the right.
To improve validity, rule out constructional and motor apraxias.

TEST NO. 1b: Copy Flower, House (Figure 4-2)[112]
Description: The therapist draws a simple flower and later a house in the presence of the patient. Each drawing is done on a fresh piece of paper, and the patient copies flower before proceeding to the house.
Scoring: Subjective.
Intact—all parts included in their proper place.
Impaired—some parts are missing from the left side (Figure 4-2) or figures are positioned too far to the right of page.
Validity: This is also a test for constructional and motor apraxias. If the patient had constructional apraxia but not unilateral neglect, he would include most of the parts but they would be jumbled and not in correct relation to each other. A patient with a dominant lesion who has constructional apraxia is helped by copying from a model. A patient with motor apraxia might have trouble doing the task at all.

TEST NO. 2: Human Figure or Face Puzzle[112]
Description: See Test No. 5 under somatognosia.
Scoring: Subjective.
Intact—all pieces correctly placed.
Impaired—pieces missing on the left side.

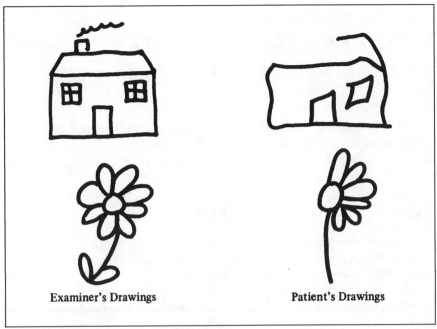

Examiner's Drawings   Patient's Drawings

Figure 4-2. Examples of impaired performance on "copy flower, house" test for unilateral neglect.

To improve validity, rule out constructional and motor apraxias (see Test No. 2 under unilateral neglect for description of qualitative differences in performance for differential diagnosis).

TEST NO. 3: Copy Pegboard Designs[112]
Description: The therapist makes up a design on a pegboard with pegs on both the left and right sides of the board. The patient is asked to copy the design exactly.
Scoring: Subjective.
Intact—all pegs correctly placed within a reasonable length of time.
Impaired—some pegs missing from design on left side.
To improve validity, rule out constructional and motor apraxias and figure-ground disorder.

TEST NO. 4: Crossing Out Letter[84,251]
Description: The therapist types random letters across several lines on a piece of paper. The patient is asked to cross out all the "A's" or whatever letter is picked (Figure 4-3).
Scoring: Nonstandardized.
Intact—all correct letters crossed out.
Impaired—letters missed on left side of page.
To improve validity, rule out poor eyesight, hemianopsia, motor apraxias.

B Ⓗ A K D O Ⓗ E L J K H̸ D E H̸ O N M C H̸ G M H̸ S J L H̸

Ⓗ I M H̸ N R W Q H̸ L O H̸ P C M B H̸ T S H̸ E W H̸ Y T R E

M G Ⓗ Y K Ⓗ G E D H̸ Y U H̸ R Q O H̸ V H̸ D C Y H̸ L E H̸ S

Errors: 5

Figure 4-3. Example of impaired performance on Crossing Out Letter test for unilateral neglect. Circled letters are the skipped letters.

TEST NO. 5: Reading[190]

Description: Ask the patient to read something aloud. Be sure to have a copy in front of you so that you can follow along with the reading.

Scoring: Subjective.

Intact—reads passage correctly without skipping words on left.

Impaired—misses words on left side of page, hesitates over beginning next line, may supply missing word to make passage coherent.

A patient showing significant impairment on this test usually has a severe unilateral neglect problem, which manifests itself in many areas of daily living.

To improve validity (not applicable with aphasics) if patient has poor eyesight, be sure to use a passage printed in large print.

TEST NO. 6: Confrontation Testing (refer to the visual neglect test in the gross visual skills section)

Treatment for Unilateral Neglect

1. Do activities that stimulate the neglected side, hoping to make the patient aware of it.
   a. Therapist rubs affected arm of patient while patient watches, using either her own hand, a rough cloth, a brush, ice, or vibrator.[3] *Caution:* check for spasticity and be careful not to increase it.
   b. Patient rubs himself with his nonaffected hand while he watches it.[3]
   c. While watching himself, patient self-ranges the affected arm and hand to assist if he has little muscle power. If patient has some proximal return, he can use a skateboard to move arm in half circles on a table, crossing the midline.[3]
2. Do activities that force the patient to look to the left so that he becomes aware of his left side and will look to the left on his own. This may work better if one uses a reinforcer like food or money.
   a. Tile work—all tiles on left side.
   b. Pegboard—all pegs on left side.[251]

---

c. Lay out coins across the table—have patient pick them up.[251]

d. Lay out numbered cards in a row in front of patient. Have him count them from right to left. Correct his mistakes. Move cards over to left side, one card space at a time, as patient correctly counts the cards. Vary the order so that activity does not become rote memorization.[190]

e. Have patient practice canceling out one letter in several lines of letters typed on a page; e.g., "Cross out all the H's that you see." If mistakes are made, tell the patient to read the letters aloud to slow him down.[84]

3. Utilizing a neurodevelopmental treatment approach, have the patient participate in bilateral tasks to facilitate increased total body awareness. Specific handling techniques and proprioceptive facilitation through weight bearing activities will also help.

4. If the patient neglects the left half of the page while reading, train him to look to the left by giving him visual guides to look for before beginning to read a line.[190]

a. A red line drawn at the left side of the page.

b. A clip-on marker.

c. His finger placed at the left side of the page.

5. Teach cognitive awareness of the problem to help the patient compensate for it.

a. Practice having the patient turn his head or shift his eyes to the left side.[190,252]

b. Have someone in the room while he is eating to give him cognitive cues and correct his errors.[252]

c. Use a mirror while dressing.[253]

d. Place a tape vertically along the floor and have the patient practice wheeling down the middle of it. Patient can visually see when he is going off course.[253]

6. When neglect causes functional problems, have the patient practice those problem areas until he does them correctly automatically; e.g., practice locking wheelchair and lifting footpedal before transferring if the patient neglects the left side. Be sure to use the same sequence of steps each practice session.[250]

7. Some adaptations:[48]

a. Put food on unaffected side.

b. Put telephone or call light on unaffected side.

c. Always speak to patient on unaffected side and stand on unaffected side.

Anosognosia

Anosognosia is a severe form of neglect to the extent that the patient fails "to recognize the presence of severity of his paralysis."[225] Anosognosia may be simply unconcern for the paralysis (anosodiaphoria) or, at the other extreme, be a complete denial of paralysis.[225] When asked whether anything is wrong, the patient denies his illness.[204] If confronted by the fact that the side is paralyzed and will not move in response to his efforts, the patient may reply that the limb has "a will and purpose of its own,"[112] that "it is tired," or that "it always was a lazy arm."

Montague Ullman[225] has attempted to interpret anosognosia as a way in which the patient experiences his body. Even transient stroke patients have described a limb as feeling "not there" or not belonging to the body. In a patient with brain damage, abstract thinking may be diminished so that he is tied to his subjective experience. Thus, if the arm does not feel a part of him or does not hurt, he cannot make reasonable judgments about it. Another variable is the patient's premorbid personality; that is, the patient may have always been one to go through life verbally denying that anything was wrong no matter what the crisis or disturbing event. With these two factors working together, the patient does not have to deal with an illness he cannot perceive, and he also separates himself from a stressful situation. In his way, he is preserving his own intactness. The following example illustrates these concepts:[225]

A patient lying in bed noticed his arm protruding from a blanket. He remarked spontaneously, "When I was put in bed, this arm was sticking out. I told the nurses and doctors. They think it's my arm, but it's not. That's been sticking out like this ever since I was put in here."

"Whose hand is it?"

"I wouldn't know. It was here when they put me in bed. I always had an idea I was laying on top of a corpse because this hand was lying out there motionless."

Anosognosia may also be a syndrome that occurs in apractognosia.

Lesion site: parietal lobe of the nondominant hemisphere, supramarginal gyrus.[60,165]

Evaluation for Anosognosia

There are no formal tests for this deficit. Some therapists use the same tests as those for unilateral neglect and say that severe impairment on these tests shows anosognosia. For example, if a patient placed the left arm and leg of the human figure puzzle off to the extreme left side of the felt board, this might be an indication that he believes that these limbs are no longer part of him. Any scoring system is extremely subjective.

Diagnosis of this deficit can usually be made by talking to the patient.

Does he realize that he is paralyzed? How does he feel about his paralysis (is he unconcerned)? Does he confabulate or rationalize about why his arm cannot move? If he denies his paralysis or says that his arm is "just a little weak," these are indications of anosognosia.

Treatment for Anosognosia

While the patient is denying his illness, it is almost impossible to teach him to compensate for it. Usually, as the patient begins to spontaneously recover, the denial disappears.

Right-Left Discrimination

A deficit in right-left discrimination causes an inability to understand and use concepts of right and left. This may be the result of personal confusion so that first the patient cannot name or point to his own right or left body parts on command, or it may be extrapersonal to the extent that the patient cannot discriminate between the examiner's right and left sides.

A deficit in right-left discrimination may also be a syndrome that occurs in apractognosia.

Lesion site: parietal lobe of either hemisphere.[165]

Evaluation for Right-Left Discrimination

TEST NO. 1: Ayres' Right-Left Discrimination Test (subtest of the Southern California Sensory Integration Tests)[14]

Description: Therapist sits facing the patient and gives the patient a series of commands.

1. Show me your right hand.
2. Touch your left ear.
3. Take this pencil with your right hand. (Hold pencil in both hands, hands resting on knees.)
4. Now put it in my right hand. (Holds hands palm up on knees.)
5. Is this pencil on your right or left side? (Hold pencil in left hand 1 foot in front of patient's right shoulder.)
6. Touch your right eye.
7. Show me your left foot.
8. Is this pencil on your right or left side? (Hold pencil in right hand in front of patient's left shoulder.)
9. Take this pencil with your left hand. (Hold pencil in both hands, hands resting on knees.)
10. Now put it in my left hand. (Hold hands palm up on knees.)

Scoring: Score 2 points if correct within three seconds and one point if correct within four to 10 seconds. If patient first makes a wrong response and then corrects himself, the score is based on the time of correct response. If the command is repeated, the score can be no more than 1. This test has been standardized only for children. In testing its reliability for children aged 4.0 to 8.11 years, the test-retest correlations ranged from r=0.15 to 0.54. Scoring for adults is nonstandardized.

Intact—as adult norms have not been established, the therapist should gather her own provisional norms by testing a few normal adults.

To improve validity, rule out aphasia and apraxia.

Reliability: Inter-rater reliability (r=0.93) was established for this test on a sample of adult head trauma patients.[23]

TEST NO. 2: Point to Body Parts on Command[203,251]

Description: The therapist asks the patient to point or indicate in some way the body parts named on himself, on the examiner, or on a human figure doll or puzzle. There is no standardized form of this test. The therapist can make up her own. For example:

1. Show me your left hand.
2. Show me your right eye.
3. Show me your left foot.
4. Show me your left shoulder.
5. Show me your right elbow.
6. Show me your left knee.
7. Show me your right ear.
8. Show me your left wrist.
9. Show me your right ankle.
10. Show me your right thumb.

Scoring: Nonstandardized.

Intact—patient correctly indicates all parts named within a reasonable length of time.

To improve validity, rule out aphasia and apraxia as causes of poor performance. This is similar to Test No. 1 under somatognosia except that the words "left" and "right" are included in the commands. The two tests could be combined by using commands with and without "left" and "right" in them. One could then compare the results. Does the patient do better with commands omitting "left" and "right"? Does he indicate the correct body part but on the wrong side, i.e., lift left hand when commanded to "Show me your right hand." Then it is a problem of right-left discrimination. If the patient is totally confused and indicates the wrong body part altogether, it may be a problem of somatognosia.

Reliability: Inter-rater reliability (r=0.94) was established for a variation of this test on a sample of adult patients with head trauma.[23]

TEST NO. 3: Orientation of Right and Left[156]

Description: Therapist sits in front of patient. The patient should·be in a position to see all four of his extremities. The therapist asks, "Am I touching you on the right or left side?" An expressive aphasic can point to previously made cards marked "right" and "left" to indicate his answer.

1. Touch the patient on the left cheek.
2. Touch the patient on the right elbow.
3. Touch the patient on the right thumb.
4. Touch the patient on the left shoulder.
5. Touch the patient on the left ankle.

Scoring: Nonstandardized.

Intact—patient answers all correctly and fairly rapidly.

To improve validity, rule out aphasia and sensory deficits.

Treatment for Right and Left Discrimination

1. Using a sensory integrative approach, give a selected hand extra tactile and proprioceptive stimulation to help patient distinguish, e.g., weighted cuff on the right wrist. Be consistent; do not switch hands.

2. Do activities that repeatedly stress right and left differences, hoping that the patient will transfer the experience.
   a. Quiz the patient about right-left discrimination; e.g., show me your left elbow; give me the right shoe.
   b. Stress right and left verbally while the patient carries out activities of daily living.[222]

3. Give the patient cognitive cues to help him compensate.
   a. The patient wears his watch on his left side in order to use his watch as a clue to help him distinguish right from left.
   b. On clothing, shoes, and so forth, mark the right side different from the left side with colored tape or a laundry pen.[48]

4. For a human environment adaptation, do not use the words "right" and "left" in commands. Either point or refer to the part by where it is located, e.g., the foot next to the bed, the affected side.[48]

Finger Agnosia

Finger agnosia consists of doubt and hesitation concerning the fingers. A fairly common occurrence, it is usually found bilaterally with more involvement of the three middle fingers of each hand. The patient has confusion in naming his fingers on command or knowing which one was touched.[112] The following describes an examination of a stroke patient for finger agnosia.[122]

It was very difficult for him (the patient) to name his own fingers on command; he frequently mixed the index and middle fingers. He seemed unable to number his fingers in any constant fashion in a given direction. When the examiner's hand was placed beside his own and he was told to copy movements, such as touching with the index finger of his other hand the same finger the examiner had touched, he did it

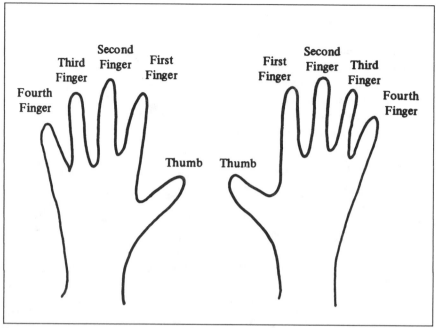

Figure 4-4. Hand chart for tests 1 and 2 under figure agnosia (reduced from life size).

accurately. However, if the examiner's hand was placed beside his in the opposite direction, he made frequent mistakes for the central fingers. When his eyes were closed, he was often inaccurate in naming the finger touched either on his right or on his left hand.

While this patient is aware of his body, he has difficulty conceiving the relationships of its different parts.[122] The patient will use his fingers hesitantly or gingerly in performing a motor task. Deficits in finger agnosia have been found to correlate highly with poor dexterity in tasks involving movement of fingers in relation to one another.

Finger agnosia frequently occurs with a group of symptoms, all of which have been called Gerstmann's syndrome. This syndrome includes finger agnosia, right-left discrimination, agraphia, and acalculia.

Lesion site: parietal lobe of the dominant hemisphere, angular gyrus.[165]

Evaluation for Finger Agnosia

TEST NO. 1: Finger Localization—Naming[156,203]

Description: Have the patient place his hands palm down on the table. A picture of two hands (Figure 4-4) is placed in front of the patient so that the fingers in the picture point in the same direction as the patient's fingers. The therapist touches the patient's fingers one at a time, saying, "I am going to touch your fingers one at a time. Name or point to the finger on the picture of the hand that is the same as the finger I touched."

This test can be given with the patient watching while he is touched and with vision occluded. A combination of both—five items with vision and five with vision occluded—is useful to compare results. To occlude vision, the therapist can ask the patient to close his eyes, or shield his eyes with a file folder, or ask the patient to place his hands in a specially made box that has two ends open, one end covered with a curtain so that the patient cannot see in. There is no standardized form of this test. The therapist can make up her own order. For example: "Which finger am I touching?" Touch the patient with a pencil eraser on his:

1. Right second finger.
2. Left third finger.
3. Right thumb.
4. Left fourth finger.
5. Right first finger.
6. Left second finger.
7. Right fourth finger.
8. Left first finger.
9. Right third finger.
10. Left first finger.

Scoring: Nonstandardized.

Intact—patient correctly indicates all fingers touched within a reasonable length of time.

To improve validity, rule out impaired sensation on both hands.

TEST NO. 2: Finger Identification by Name[156,203]

Description: The patient is asked to move or point to the finger on his own hand named by the therapist. A variation of this test is to have the patient point to the finger on his hand matching the one the therapist points to on the hand chart (Figure 4-4). This test is not standardized. The therapist can make up her own order. Five to 10 commands is probably sufficient. For example see Test No. 1 under finger agnosia.

Scoring: Nonstandardized.

Intact—patient correctly indicates all fingers named within a reasonable length of time.

To improve validity, rule out aphasia.

TEST NO. 3: Imitation[203]

Description: Patient is instructed to imitate finger movements made by the therapist. There is no standardized form of this test. The therapist can make up her own movements. Five movements are sufficient. For example:

1. Therapist curls right index finger forward.
2. Therapist touches left thumb to tip of left little finger.
3. Therapist touches left middle finger with tip of right index finger.
4. Therapist brings left index and middle fingers together laterally.
5. Therapist circumducts right thumb.

Scoring: Subjective.

Intact—patient imitates all movements correctly within a reasonable length of time.

To improve validity, rule out apraxia and paralysis/paresis of affected hand.

Treatment for Finger Agnosia

Both sensorimotor and transfer of training treatment approaches have been used with success in this area.[93]

1. Applying the sensory integrative approach to treating finger agnosia, Julia Fox[93] recommended stimulating the patient's discriminative tactile system's touch and pressure receptors by (1) rubbing vigorously the dorsal surface of the affected forearm, hand, and fingers and the ventral surface of the affected fingers with a rough cloth, and (2) applying pressure to the ventral surface of the hand by asking the patient to grasp a cardboard cone, either actively or passively. Each type of stimulation should be done for a minimum of two minutes though one can alternate: 30 seconds rubbing, 30 seconds pressure. The patient should be told that the treatment should feel good and to tell the therapist when it feels uncomfortable. Be on the alert for signs of discomfort, such as a slight withdrawal response when stroking the fingers. When this happens, change the stimulation to a new area to avoid activation of the protective response.

2. Believing improvement on one task will transfer to similar tasks, quiz the patient on finger identification; e.g., show me or touch your right index finger.

CHAPTER V

Spatial Relations Syndrome

The spatial relations syndrome, an important area of perceptual problems, includes defects common to two types of apraxia and agnosia. This syndrome presents varied problems in perceiving spatial relationships and distances between objects or between self and two or more objects. This syndrome occurs most frequently with right-sided brain lesions and includes the following disabilities: figure ground, form constancy, position in space, spatial relations, constructional apraxia, dressing apraxia, topographical disorientation, and depth and distance perceptual deficits.

Figure Ground

The patient has trouble differentiating the foreground from the background. The "figure" or foreground is the part of the field of perception that is the center of an individual's attention at any given time. Those incoming stimuli that are not the center of attention form the dimly perceived background.[98] A figure-ground deficit often leads to a short attention span because the patient is easily distracted.[115] He may have trouble finding things, for instance, his hairbrush in a cluttered drawer or the sleeve of his all-white shirt.

Lesion site: parietal lobe of nondominant hemisphere[165] and a large lesion or many small lesions anywhere in the brain.[12]

Evaluation for Figure Ground

TEST NO. 1: Ayres' Figure-Ground Test (subtest of the Southern California Sensory Integration Tests)[14]

Description: This is a published test requiring the patient to select three pictures of objects or geometric forms from a multiple choice plate of six pictures. The three to be selected are to be found in an embedded plate (Figure 5-1). The patient indicates his choice by naming or pointing to the picture or design. He has one minute to identify three embedded pictures. The test is discontinued after five errors.

Scoring: Each correctly identified picture is given a score of 1. The range of possible scores is 0 to 48.

This test has been standardized only for children up to the age of 10.11 years. A score of 18 is the mean for 10.11 year olds. However, a pilot normative study was done at Boston University[158] with normal adults aged 20 to 59 with the following results:

Age	Number of Subjects	Mean Score	One Standard Deviation
20-29	22	31.9	9.7
30-39	12	32.6	8.9
40-49	10	22.8	7.8
50-59	12	23.9	5.7

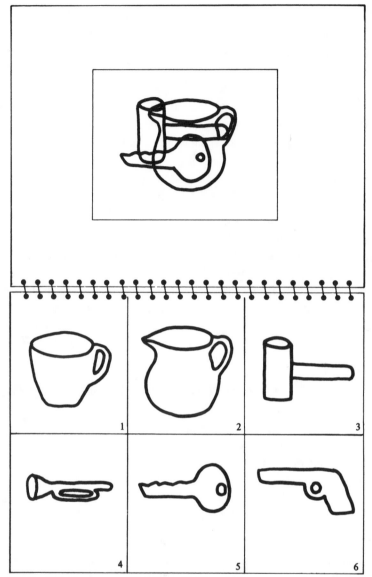

Figure 5-1. One page of Southern California figure ground perception test.

However, until a more extensive normative study can be done, interpretation of scores for this test for adults is nonstandardized.

Intact—one standard deviation ($\pm$).

Impaired—more than minus 1 standard deviation from the mean.

Severely impaired—more than minus 2 standard deviations from the mean.

Validity: Rule out poor eyesight, hemianopsia, and dense aphasia. (For mild aphasics who understand gestures, the test may be valid.) This test has been found to discriminate between children with and without perceptual deficits ($t = 5.19$, $p<0.01$). Its reliability test-retest coefficients of correlation range from $r=0.37$ to 0.52 for children aged 4.0 to 10.11 years.

Reliability: This test has established inter-rater reliability (r=0.87) on a sample of adult patients with head trauma.[23]

This test requires a high degree of concentration. Therefore, it may not be valid to administer it to patients who show a high degree of distractibility.

TEST NO. 2: Frostig Figure Ground

Description: This is a published subtest of the Frostig Developmental Test of Visual Perception.[97] The patient is asked to outline several embedded geometric shapes with a colored pencil. The number of distractors increases with each item.

Scoring: Frostig's test has been standardized only for children. In testing its reliability in 127 kindergarteners and first graders, the test-retest correlations ranged from r = 0.42 to 0.46.[99] Scoring for adults is nonstandardized.

Intact—patient outlines figure without starting to outline another figure.

Factors affecting validity: This test overlaps with eye-hand coordination, motor praxias, visual acuity, and abstract concepts.

Reliability: In a study conducted in adult patients who sustained head trauma, this test showed a negative correlation with the remaining figure ground tests.[23] The Frostig figure ground test, however, showed a significant correlation ($p<0.01$) with the constructional praxis subtest. These results indicate that the test was measuring constructional abilities rather than figure ground skills. Further research may indicate that this test is not an appropriate test for the adult patient with brain damage. If this is the case, it is recommended that the test be deleted from the perceptual evaluation.

TEST NO. 3: Functional Test[250,251,255]

Descripton: The therapist asks the patient to pick out or find an object in view. There are many variations of this test. Here are some examples:

1. While in the patient's bedroom, ask the patient to pick up a white towel or face cloth that you have put on his white sheets.

2. While dressing, ask the patient to find his sleeve, buttonholes, buttons, and bottom of the shirt.

3. While in the kitchen, ask the patient to find objects that are on the counter or the knife among the unsorted cutlery in the drawer.

4. Ask the patient to sort a pile of shirts into long and short sleeved.

Scoring: Subjective.

Intact—patient does tasks within a reasonable length of time.

To improve validity, rule out poor eyesight, visual object agnosia and poor comprehension of the directions as reasons for poor performance.

Treatment for Figure Ground

1. Believing that improvement in one task will transfer to similar tasks, scatter 10 objects in a disorganized fashion in front of the patient. Name an object and have the patient point to it. Increase the

number of objects as the patient improves. To use with aphasics, have ready a second set of identical objects. Show the patient the object you want him to find.[222]

2. When this deficit causes functional problems, the patient should practice the problem areas until he does them correctly automatically; e.g., if the patient has difficulty finding the wheelchair brake, practice locking and unlocking the chair while practicing transferring.[250]

3. To help the patient compensate, teach him cognitive awareness of his deficit; teach him to be very systematic and examine each small area carefully by slowing down and not being impulsive. For example, in the kitchen, have him look and even feel the counter top to find out what objects are on it.[255]

4. Adapt the environment, make it simple and uncluttered.[48,255]

    a. Put only a few things on the night stand.

    b. Organize drawers, separating articles.

    c. Arrange the meal tray so that it has only a few items; have the meal in several courses if necessary.

    d. Mark the wheelchair brakes with red tape so that they will be easier to distinguish from wheel.

Form Constancy

This disorder involves an inability to attend to subtle variations in form to the extent that the patient may confuse his water pitcher and his urinal since they have similar shapes.

Lesion site: parietal lobe of nondominant hemisphere.[165]

Evaluation for Form Constancy

TEST NO. 1: Frostig Form Constancy

Description: This is a published subtest of the Frostig Developmental Test of Visual Perception.[97] The patient is asked to trace around all the squares and circles he can find on the page. He is shown a line drawing of a square and circle to aid in comprehension. The page has many confusing figures and similar shapes.

Scoring: Frostig's test has been standardized only for children. In testing its reliability in 127 kindergarteners and first graders, the test-retest correlations ranged from $r = 0.67$ to 0.83.[99] Scoring for adults is nonstandardized.

Intact—patient correctly traces around all squares and circles.

To improve validity, rule out figure ground problems and poor eye-hand coordination, especially if the patient is using nondominant hand. Rule out poor eyesight and hemianopsia.

TEST NO. 2: Functional Test

Description: Collect a group of similar objects of different sizes behind a screen, e.g., small and large combs or mugs. Present them one at a time to the patient and ask him to identify them. Present each object several times but in different positions and sizes each time, e.g., upside down, at right angles.

Scoring: Subjective.

Intact—patient correctly identifies most of objects within a reasonable length of time.

To improve validity, rule out aphasia and visual object agnosia.

TEST NO. 3: Formboard Test*.[247]

Procedure: Show the patient the 10 forms and test plate. Hand the patient one form at a time, telling him to match each shape on the boards. The therapist may give a demonstration for aphasic patients. Take the form away after the patient has matched it, out of eyesight, so that he cannot use the process of elimination.

Directions: "Place each form on the shape that matches it."

Observe for spatial neglect, perseveration, poor planning or comprehension, and general inability to deal with objects.

Score:

Severely impaired—unable to match more than one to four forms.

Impaired—able to match five to nine forms.

Intact—matches all 10 forms correctly.

To improve validity, rule out poor vision, visual field loss, poor color discrimination, and constructional apraxia as causes of poor performance.

Reliability: Inter-rater reliability (r=1.0) was established for this test on a sample of adult patients with head trauma.[23]

Treatment for Form Constancy

1. Believing improvement in one task will transfer to similar tasks, have the patient practice various tasks in which he must discriminate subtle variations in form. For example:

   a. Have the patient match similar parquetry blocks to each other. Call attention to errors as they are made.[252]

   b. Have the patient sort a pile of clothes by category, e.g., pants, shorts, long and short sleeve shirts. Discuss with the patient the discriminating cues he used to separate clothing.[222]

   c. Present the same object in various positions and sizes and ask the patient to identify it. A variation of this is to have several similarly shaped objects behind a screen and pres-

---

* Reproduced with permission from Santa Clara Valley Medical Center, San Jose, California.

ent them one at a time to the patient to identify verbally or by demonstration of its use. If one uses this treatment idea, do not use the Functional Test No. 2 to retest the patient as it will no longer be a valid test.
d. Type a row of letters using both capitals and small letters. Have patient find all the A's (a's) (verbalized "A's"). For example:

A B b C c K a J H A R u i V B a L o p U V A b C

e. Utilize computer activities that focus on form discrimination.

Position in Space

Impaired position in space is the inability to interpret and deal with concepts of spatial positioning of objects, such as in-out, up-down, front-behind. For example, if told the waste basket was under the desk, the patient might not know where to look for it.

Lesion site: parietal lobe of the nondominant hemisphere.[165]

Evaluation for Position in Space

TEST NO. 1: Frostig Position in Space

Description: This is a published subtest of the Frostig Developmental Test of Visual Perception.[97] The test consists of two parts with four items each. In Part A the patient is asked to look at a row of line drawings and find the one that is different from the others. The difference is always a rotational transformation one. In Part B the patient is asked to look at a row of similar line drawings and find one that is the same as the drawing in the left hand margin. Again the only difference is a rotational one.

Modifications: Many clinics have made up their own versions of this test on felt cards. For example, one clinic used felt cards with four identical flowers, one of which was upside down. The patient was asked to find one that was different.[250,251]

Scoring: Frostig's test has been standardized only for children ages four to eight. In testing its reliability in 127 kindergarteners and first graders, the test-retest correlation ranged from r=0.61 to 0.63.[99] Scoring for adults is nonstandardized.

Intact—patient identifies all items correctly.

To improve validity, rule out incomprehension of the directions owing to aphasia or not knowing what is meant by the concepts "similar" and "different." Rule out poor eyesight.

Reliability: In a study of adult head trauma patients, this test did not reach an acceptable level of inter-rater reliability (r=0.70).[23] In addition, item analysis indicated a low correlation between this test and the Southern California Sensory Integration Tests.

Additional research is indicated to justify the use of the Frostig Position in Space Test with the adult brain damaged population.

78

TEST NO. 2: Positioning Blocks

Description: The therapist places two small cube blocks in front of the patient and asks him to place one block in various positions in relation to the other block, e.g., on top, behind, in front of, to the right, to the left. There is no standardized form of this test. The therapist makes up her own commands.

Scoring: Subjective.

Intact—patient correctly does each move within a reasonable length of time.

To improve validity, rule out aphasia and apraxia.

Reliability: In a study of adult patients with head trauma, all 20 subjects scored intact on a variation of this test.[23] Further research should indicate whether this test discriminates well for the adult brain damaged population.

TEST NO. 3: Two-Dimensional Drawings[251]

Description: Use several cards with pictures of the same two objects drawn or pasted on each one. One object should be placed in a different position in relation to the other object on each card. For example, a series of cards might have a shoe and a box on each card with the shoe placed to the right, the left, above, or beneath the box, depending on the card. Place the cards in a line in front of the patient and ask him to find, in turn, the card where the shoe is to the right, the left, above, or beneath the box.

Scoring: Subjective.

Intact—patient correctly finds each card asked for within a reasonable length of time.

To improve validity, rule out figure ground problems, hemianopsia, unilateral neglect, and aphasia as causes of poor performance.

Validity of Tests No. 2 and No. 3: Tests No. 2 and No. 3 are really testing the patient's knowledge of the concepts on top, behind, above, beneath, right, and left, which are more abstract ideas than may be necessary for the patient to know his position in space. The correlation between the tests and the patient's functional use of position in space has not been examined.

TEST NO. 4: Ayres' Position in Space Test (subtest of Southern California Sensory Integration Tests)[14]

Description: This test measures the perception of the same form (or forms) in different orientations. It is a 30-item test divided into three parts, each part measuring a slightly different aspect. Part 3 measures memory of position in space. To use the test as a discrete test of position in space, it is recommended that one use only Parts 1 and 2.

Scoring: This test has been standardized for children aged 4.0 to 10.11 years. In testing its reliability, the test-retest correlations ranged from $r = 0.33$ to 0.78. This test is nonstandardized for adults. In a pilot normative study done at Boston University[158] with adults aged 20 to 49, all the subjects scored perfectly on the first two parts of the test. All of the errors occurred in the third part of the test. Therefore, we can tentatively say that a normal adult should complete all items on Parts 1 and 2 correctly.

To improve validity, rule out incomprehension of the directions, poor eyesight.

Reliability: Inter-rater reliability (r=0.89) was established for this test in a study of adult patients with head trauma.[23]

TEST NO. 5: Felt Pictures[251]

Description: The therapist shows the patient a felt card with identical pictures on both halves of the card, except that the right side has one object missing. The patient is asked to place that object (a felt cut-out shape) on the card so that the two pictures are identical. There is no standardized form of this test. Each therapist can make up her own cards. Here are some examples:

1. House and tree—the patient has to place the tree in the same relation to the house as in the copy on the left.

2. Shirt and shirt pocket—the patient has to place the shirt pocket in the same place as on the shirt in the copy on the left.

3. Shirt and tie—the patient has to place the tie in the same position as in the copy on the left.

Scoring: Subjective.

Intact—patient does task correctly without hesitation.

To improve validity, rule out figure ground, motor apraxia, poor eye-hand coordination.

Treatment for Position in Space

1. Believing improvement in one task will transfer to similar tasks, have the patient practice various tasks in which he must discriminate different orientations in space. For example:

   a. Place four cardboard squares in front of the patient. Ask him to place them parallel so that the sides are horizontal and vertical.

   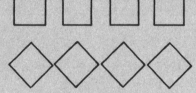

   Scatter them and ask the patient to turn them so that they all stand on a corner.

Repeat this procedure with triangles.[98]

   b. Use several cards, each with a row of identical figures, one of which is upside down in relation to the others. Ask the patient to find the one figure that is different on each card. Discuss his errors.

   c. Using two 1 inch cube blocks, the patient practices placing one block on top, in front, behind, to the right, and to the left of the other block in response to your command. Discuss his errors.

Spatial Relations

The patient has trouble perceiving the position of two or more objects in relation to himself and in relation to each other. For example, a child stringing beads in a certain sequence has to perceive the position of the bead and the string in relation to himself as well as the position of the beads and the string in relation to each other.[99]

Refer to this subject also under apractognosia and visual spatial agnosia.

Lesion site: parietal lobe of the nondominant hemisphere.[51]

Evaluation of Spatial Relations

TEST NO. 1: Frostig Spatial Relations

Description: This is a published subtest of the Frostig Developmental Test of Visual Perception.[97] On one half of the page is a matrix of dots with lines drawn through them to form a pattern. On the other half of the page is just a matrix of dots. The patient is asked to connect the dots so that they form the same pattern as the one on the left side of the page.

Scoring: Frostig's test has been standardized only for children ages four to eight. In testing its reliability in 127 kindergarteners and first graders, the test-retest correlations ranged from $r=0.59$ to 0.66. Scoring for adults is subjective.

Intact—all patterns correctly done.

To improve validity, rule out unilateral neglect, hemianopsia, figure ground problems, poor eye-hand coordination, constructional apraxia, and perseveration as causes of poor performance. Some therapists use this test as an organization task. They watch how the patient goes about doing the task.

TEST NO. 2: Cross Test[186]

Description: This test requires the patient to duplicate a small cross on a blank sheet of paper in the same position as it appeared on the stimulus card (Figure 5-2). A blank piece of paper, the sample stimulus card, and a black felt pen are placed in front of the patient, and he is instructed to "Draw two small crosses on this paper in the exact positions that they appeared on the card. Be exact." If the patient does not understand, the therapist demonstrates by drawing the crosses for him. After the patient does the sample, the transparent score guide is placed over the trial so that the patient can judge the extent of his discrepancies. Then each of the three test cards is presented in turn, with the command, "Now do the same thing with this card. Place a cross in the same position on this sheet of paper as it is on the test card. Do not hurry. Be exact."

Scoring: Nonstandardized. The subject's score is the total number of centimeters of discrepancy between the model and the reproduction. The transparent score guide is placed over the subject's effort, and the distances between the intersection of lines on the model and the subject's crosses are measured with a centimeter ruler. If there is any doubt as to which cross the patient was attempting to copy, the model closest to

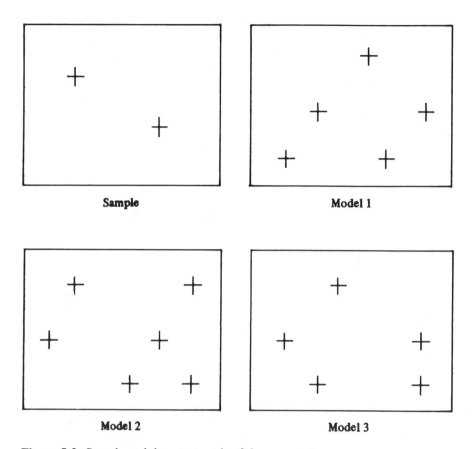

Figure 5-2. Sample and three test cards of the cross test.

his cross should be selected. If a cross is missing from a patient's effort, this should be scored as one-half the width of the page.

Intact—score of 0 to 300.

Impaired—score of 300 to 600.

Severe—score of 600 and above. (Scores adapted from those received by control group in study of Pehoski.[186])

To improve validity, rule out motor apraxia, poor eye-hand coordination, unilateral neglect, and hemianopsia.

TEST NO. 3: Ayres' Space Visualization Test (subtest of Southern California Sensory Integration Tests[14])

Description: This test uses two formboards, one with an egg-shaped hollow and one with a diamond-shaped hollow, two pegs, four egg-shaped blocks, and four diamond-shaped blocks. The pegs are inserted into the formboards to create different test items. The tests consist of 30 "puzzles," each consisting of one formboard and two blocks, only one of which fits the formboard. The patient is asked to look at the puzzle and choose one of the two blocks. Only then is he allowed to try fitting his choice in the formboard. The test is discontinued after five errors are made.

82

Scoring: This test has been standardized only for children. In testing the reliability, Ayres reports the test-retest correlations range from r=0.28 to 0.77 for children aged 4.0 to 10.11 years.

Using the same scoring method as Ayres, Taylor[221] provides the following normative data:

	Age	Number of Subjects	Mean Score	Standard Deviation
Accuracy	50-64	90	56.2	4.5
	65-74	60	56.3	4.5
Time	50-64	90	118.2	50.8
	65-74	60	158.5	74.9

However, until a more extensive normative study can be done, interpretation of scores is nonstandardized.

Intact—one standard deviation.

Impaired—more than minus 1 standard deviation from the mean.

Validity: Ayres[11] reported a study in which she administered this test to both right and left hemiplegic adults. The left hemiplegics did better as a group than the right hemiplegics, although the difference was not significant. Because generally it is thought that left hemiplegics do significantly poorer on spatial relations tests, the validity of this test with adults is in some doubt.

TEST NO. 4: The Bender Visual Motor Gestalt Test[183]

Description: The patient is given a piece of 8½ × 11 inch plain paper and a pencil. He is shown nine cards, one at a time, and asked to draw the design he sees on each card. He draws all nine designs on the one piece of paper.

Scoring: Standardized. In testing its reliability, the authors report a test-retest correlation of r=0.71 and a score reliability of r=0.90. This test has elaborate directions for scoring. To learn how to score it, one must consult the manual.

Validity: This test has been used diagnostically with many different populations: brain-damaged, psychotic, delinquent, and normal children and adults. Rule out unilateral neglect, hemianopsia, poor eyesight, and poor coordination due to paresis or use of the nondominant hand.

Treatment of Spatial Relations

In the belief that improvement in one task will transfer to similar tasks, have the patient practice tasks in which he must orient himself to two or more objects. And believing that there is a developmental sequence in learning perceptual skills, first have the patient practice tasks in which he has to orient himself to space and then proceed with object to object orientation. As an example of patient orienting himself to space: Make a furniture maze in the treatment room. Either draw a map or just ask the patient to go from point A to point B. This can be used with both ambulatory and wheelchair patients. With some patients, one could incorporate rewards, e.g., find the treasure hidden here—treasure map idea. Remember, though, that using a map requires the patient to revisualize or orient an object to space and is therefore a harder task.[222,255] An example of object to object orientation is to have the patient practice various copying tasks. Help him learn visual cues to cognitively do the task. Start with simple figures and then use more complex ones; first three-dimensional objects and then pictures. Continue when the patient successfully completes simpler tasks.

    a. Block designs—can use designs in Frostig's teacher's guide, KOH block designs on WAIS or WISC, or parquetry block designs; patient copies arrangement done by therapist.[3]

    b. Matchstick design—patient copies arrangement done by therapist.[3]

    c. Pegboards—patient copies pattern done by therapist.[3,251]

    d. Connecting dots—use designs in Frostig workbook.[3]

    e. Patient converts a two-dimensional paper pattern to a three-dimensional one using a pegboard, blocks, or parquetry blocks.[2]

    f. Puzzles—start with large four-piece puzzles. The subject of the puzzle should be a single object familiar to the patient—a person or an article of daily use.[3,251]

Constructional Apraxia

Constructional apraxia is an impairment in producing designs in two or three dimensions, by copying, drawing, or constructing, whether upon command or spontaneously. In drawing or constructing, patients with this difficulty appear to have great trouble with perspective; thus, the pieces of the composition tend to be scattered about without proper relationships to one another. (For a full description, evaluation, and treatment, refer to this topic under apraxia.)

Lesion site: occipitoparietal lobe of either hemisphere.[165]

Dressing Apraxia

Dressing apraxia is a difficulty in dressing, to the extent that the patient may not be able to relate the articles of clothing to his body or may not be able to relate parts of clothes to each other. (For full description, evaluation and treatment, refer to this topic under apraxia.)

Lesion site: occipitoparietal lobe, more often of the nondominant hemisphere.[165]

Topographical Disorientation

The patient has difficulty in understanding and remembering relationships of places to one another so that he may have difficulty in finding his way in space. (Also refer to this under apractognosia and visual spatial agnosia.)

Lesion site: occipitoparietal lobe of nondominant hemisphere.[155]

Evaluation of Topographical Disorientation

Generally the test for this deficit is a functional one. If the patient is unable to find his way back to his ward from the treatment room or from occupational therapy to physical therapy after being shown several times, this suggests a topographical disorientation problem. However, one must first rule out a general poor memory problem or mental confusion. Usually topographical disorientation is not seen in isolation from the other problems in the spatial relations syndrome. A patient without these other problems is probably "getting lost" for another reason.

Another way to test this deficit, especially if the patient is not wheeling himself to and from therapy, is to ask him to draw the route he would use to get from one specified room to another on a floor plan of his house (one will need the cooperation of the patient's relatives to obtain a floor plan). This evaluation idea is untested. It may be too abstract for some stroke patients.

Treatment for Topographical Disorientation

1. Believing improvement in one task will transfer to similar tasks, have the patient practice tasks in which he has to get from one place to another. For example, if the rehabilitation department is laid out so that this is practical, have the patient practice getting from occupational therapy to physical therapy just following verbal directions. Try simple routes and then more complicated ones. Or have the patient find his way to a designated place in occupational therapy.[250]

2. To help the patient compensate for his deficit, place him in one environment and have him learn it by rote memorization. Teach

him safety rules (such as do not go out by yourself, do not drive) and explain the reason for the rules.[255]

3. One way to adapt the patient's environment is to use markers like colored dots to mark a route the patient must travel every day. Eventually, the patient may memorize the route and one may gradually remove the cues.[255]

Depth and Distance Perceptual Deficits

The patient misjudges depths and distances so that he may have difficulty navigating stairs and architectural barriers.[115] (Refer to visual spatial agnosia.)

Evaluation for Depth and Distance Perceptual Deficits

TEST NO. 1: Blocks[251]

Description: The therapist lines up a row of small cube blocks so that they are lined perpendicular to the patient. The patient is asked in turn, "Which block is nearest?" "Which block is farthest away?" and "Which block is in the middle?" The questions are repeated after the therapist has moved the blocks so that they are lined up diagonally to the patient.

Scoring: Subjective.

Intact—patient correctly identifies each block asked for.

To improve validity, rule out aphasia. Make sure the patient understands the concepts "nearest," "farthest away," and "in the middle."

Reliability: In a study of adult patients with head trauma, there was no variance in performance on this test (i.e., all subjects scored intact).[23] This test therefore may be a poor discriminator for the adult patient with brain damage.

TEST NO. 2: Functional Test[251]

Description: Put a pen on the table in front of the patient. Ask him to grasp it. Hold the pen in the air in front of the patient. Ask him to take it from you. Ask patient to pour water from a pitcher into a glass. Ask him to position his wheelchair for a transfer.

Scoring: Subjective.

Intact—patient correctly does each request without hesitation.

To improve validity, rule out apraxia, poor eye-hand coordination, poor visual acuity, unilateral neglect, and hemianopsia.

Reliability: In a refined version of this test in a study of adult head trauma patients, 90 percent scored intact, indicating little variance in performance.[23] Additional research should indicate whether the test is appropriate for use with the adult patient with brain damage.

TEST NO. 3: Instructo Clinic—Depth Perception Test[131]

Description: The patient stands 20 feet away from the testing apparatus, which contains three road signs (stop, yield, and railroad crossing). The patient views four picture sets and is asked to tell which sign is nearest and which is farthest away.

Scoring: Nonstandardized.

The number of correct responses is calculated and divided into categories of good, satisfactory, and marginal.

To improve validity, rule out aphasia, visual field, and other visual deficits (i.e., blurred, double vision) as causes of poor performance.

Treatment for Depth and Distance Perceptual Deficits

1. The patient should be made aware of his deficit and alerted to move more cautiously, especially when navigating stairs.

2. Believing that improvement in one task will transfer to similar tasks, have the patient practice tasks in which he must judge depth and distances. If the tasks practiced are functional ones that the patient can use in daily living, so much the better. For example:

   a. In walking up and down stairs, have the patient practice feeling a high and low step by moving his foot slowly along the different step heights.

   b. If the patient is ambulatory, make a furniture maze in the treatment room. Include pieces of wood that the patient must walk over and overhead slings that he must walk under. Ask the patient to walk from point A to point B or draw a map for him to follow. For patients with whom it is appropriate, rewards can be incorporated, e.g., a treasure map with a hidden treasure to find.

   c. After trying to visually determine distances, the patient can test his answers by the counting of steps he needed to cover the distances to see which ones were actually closer or farther away.

   d. If tactile sensation in the fingers is intact, have the patient practice pouring by putting his finger near the inside top of a glass to feel when he has poured a full glass.

CHAPTER VI

The Agnosias

Agnosia, the area of perceptual deficits that deals with the patient's lack of recognition of familiar objects perceived by the senses, occurs frequently in patients who sustain strokes. It may involve a disturbance in one or all of the following sensory modes—visual, tactile, proprioceptive, and auditory—or may involve additional problems in body scheme, such as somatognosia or anosognosia.

Visual Agnosia

Visual agnosia is caused by a disturbance in the visual association area of the cortex. It includes both visual object agnosia and visual spatial agnosia.

Visual Object Agnosia

Visual object agnosia is the inability to recognize objects, although visual acuity and the ability to recognize objects by touch are still intact.[112] Visual "stimuli pass through the eye and optic tracts normally, but are not interpreted correctly in the occipital cortex."[147] These patients can fail to recognize their relatives or their possessions. The following are types of visual object agnosia that may occur separately or together: simultanognosia, prosopagnosia, color agnosia, and metamorphopsia.

Lesion site: occipitotemporoparietal lobes of either hemisphere.[112,165]

Simultanognosia. This disorder involves impairment in interpreting a visual stimulus as a whole. It seems to result from an "extreme reduction in visual span of apprehension."[229] Given a whole picture, the patient absorbs only one aspect or part at a time. For instance, a patient could point out individual letters or features, but cannot give an accurate account of the whole word.[231]

Lesion site: occipitoparietal lobe of the dominant hemisphere.[165,231]

Prosopagnosia. Prosopagnosia is the inability to recognize differences in faces. Patients with lesions in the right hemisphere "are impaired relative to left hemisphere lesioned patients in recognizing well known faces and in the immediate memory of unknown faces."[230] DeRenzi and Spinnler[81] have concluded that this defect is one of "subtle discrimination and integration of visuo-perceptive data and not an incapacity for grasping individuality within a category." These patients are able to recognize a face as a face and see differences in faces, but are not able to connect the face with recognizing someone.[230] The following excerpts are taken from an examination of a stroke patient for prosopagnosia:[122]

He complained spontaneously that he could not recognize people: "I don't recognize anybody till I have seen them a long time." He stated that he knew he had seen someone before but he was unable to make the connection between a person's name and face. . . . He knew that there are differences in faces and could not explain his trouble; certainly, faces were not distorted. He knew himself perfectly when looking in a mirror. . . . Pictures of political figures which, as he said himself, are constantly in the news were not identified, save that of Mrs. Roosevelt, and even then he could not give any verbal description of it. . . . Pictures of animals were easily recognized. He said he could visualize clearly his wife's face but not other people's. He could only imagine certain traits, such as a mustache or a bald head, but not for the over-all features.

Lesion site: parietal lobe of nondominant hemisphere.[165]

Color Agnosia. Color agnosia is the inability to recognize colors such that the patient cannot pick out a color or name a color on command.[122] This patient should be able to say whether two colors are the same or different if visual sensation is still intact. Color agnosia appears to occur more commonly after left hemisphere lesions.

Lesion site: occipital lobe of either hemisphere, but more frequently in the dominant one.[165]

Metamorphopsia. Metamorphopsia is a visual distortion of objects, although the object may be recognized accurately. For instance, a chair may appear larger or smaller than it actually is.

Lesion site: temporal lobe of the nondominant hemisphere.[165]

Evaluation of Visual Object Agnosia

TEST NO. 1: Object Recognition[251]

Description: Place several common objects in front of the patient, e.g., comb, glass, key, pencil, coin, and toothbrush. Ask him to pick up the object named and either demonstrate or tell you its functional use. There is no standardized form for this test.

Scoring: Subjective.

Intact—patient correctly identifies all objects within a reasonable length of time. To improve validity, rule out receptive aphasia, apraxia.

Treatment of Visual Object Agnosia

1. Believing that patients can relearn to recognize objects and people, give the patient discrimination drills. For example:

   a. Using photographs, have the patient try to memorize the names of faces of people important to him, e.g., his family, his doctor and nurse. Help him pick out cues for connecting faces to names.

   b. Using color cards, drill the patient in the names of colors. Start by having him discriminate between and name only two colors; gradually increase the number as he improves.

2. To help the patient compensate, encourage him to use whatever sensory mode is still intact. If he can recognize objects by touch but not by sight, tell him to feel objects.

Visual Spatial Agnosia

Visual spatial agnosia is the deficit in perceiving spatial relationships between objects or between objects and self, independently of visual object agnosia. This syndrome includes the following difficulties:

1. Spatial relations syndrome. See this under its own title for a complete description.

2. Lack of spatial orientation such that the patient cannot orient himself or objects in space. He may often be lost in his surroundings.*,[122]

3. Loss of topographical orientation such that the patient cannot understand relationships of places to one another.

4. Loss of topographical memory such that the patient cannot remember familiar routes from one place to another.

5. Difficulty in judging distances so that the patient may go to sit in a chair and misjudge so that he misses the chair.

6. Difficulty in depth perception so that the patient may continue pouring water into a glass after it is filled.

Lesion site: parietal lobe of either hemisphere.[165]

Evaluation and Treatment for Visual Spatial Agnosia

Evaluation and treatment for the foregoing symptoms may be found under the Spatial Relations Syndrome on the following pages: (1) spatial relations, page 81, (2) topographical disorientation, page 85, and (3) distance and depth perception, page 86.

Tactile Agnosia

Tactile agnosia, or astereognosis, is the inability to recognize objects or forms by handling, although tactile, thermal, and proprioceptive functions are still intact. With vision occluded, the patient is unable to recognize a key or spool of thread by touch. Related to tactile agnosia is morphognosia, the inability to tactily recognize two-dimensional shapes with vision occluded. Also included under this heading is ahylognosia, the inability to differentiate between qualities of materials, for example, between rough and fine sandpaper.[204] The therapist should be aware that in evaluating for tactile agnosia, the tests utilize the patient's capacity for multimodal input and interpretation, abstract visualization, and language function.

Lesion site: parietal lobes of either hemisphere.[112,211]

Evaluation for Tactile Agnosia

TEST NO. 1: Stereognosis[93,112]

Description: Tell the patient, "I am going to put a form like one of these in your hand so that you can feel it for a little while. Then I'll show you all the forms and you

---

*This reference is a source of extensive information about visual spatial agnosia.

can show me the one that was in your hand." Demonstrate by putting one of the objects in the patient's hand and have him feel it. Then put it back in the tray and have him show you which object he felt. Occlude the patient's vision by having him close his eyes, shield them with a file folder, or use a box like the one described in Test No. 1 under finger agnosia. Be sure that the patient does not drop objects onto the table and get auditory cues, e.g., by running finger along teeth of comb. Common objects often used for this test are a ball, spoon, pencil, key, penny, ring, button, block, and scissors. Test each hand alternately.

Scoring: Nonstandardized.

Intact—patient correctly identifies all objects within a reasonable length of time.

To improve validity, rule out impaired tactile sensation and paresis in the affected hand so that the patient cannot feel or move the object around to feel its shape. Rule out impaired sensation in nonaffected hand.

TEST NO. 2: Ayres' Manual Form Perception (subtest of Southern California Sensory Integration Tests)[14]

Description: Procedure is the same as Test No. 1. Objects used are 10 plastic geometric forms, e.g., oval, triangle, circle, star, square, hexagon, octagon, diamond, cross, and trapezoid. The object is placed in the patient's hand while his vision is occluded by a file folder shield. The patient is asked to identify the object he is feeling from 12 geometric forms printed on a piece of cardboard placed before him. Hands are tested alternately. Bilateral manipulation of form is not allowed.

Scoring: This test has been standardized for children aged 4.0 to 8.11 years. In testing reliability, Ayres reports that the test-retest correlations range from $r=0.20$ to 0.64. Scoring for adults is nonstandardized.

Intact—patient correctly identifies all 10 forms within a reasonable length of time.

To improve validity, rule out impaired tactile sensation and paresis of the affected hand and impaired sensation of the nonaffected hand.

TEST NO. 3: Morphognosis

Description: Same as test for stereognosis except that one uses geometric shapes cut out of stiff paper, only $\frac{1}{32}$ inch thick, instead of three-dimensional objects. Common shapes used are a diamond, circle, triangle, octagon, square, and egg shape.

Scoring: Nonstandardized.

Intact—patient correctly identifies all shapes within a reasonable length of time.

To improve validity, rule out lack of tactile sensation and paresis of the affected hand and impaired sensation of the nonaffected hand.

TEST NO. 4: Ahylognosis

Description: Same as test for stereognosis except that one uses materials of different textures. Some common materials used are rough and fine sandpaper, silk, plastic wrap, terrycloth, and corduroy.

Scoring: Nonstandardized.

Intact—patient correctly identifies all textures within a reasonable length of time.

To improve validity, rule out impaired tactile sensation and paresis of the affected hand and impaired sensation of the nonaffected hand.

Treatment of Tactile Agnosia

1. Adapting the sensory integrative approach, Julia Fox[93] recommended stimulating the patient's discriminative tactile system's touch and pressure receptors by (1) vigorously rubbing the dorsal surface of the affected forearm, hand, fingers, and the ventral surface of the affected fingers with a rough cloth, and (2) applying pressure to the ventral surface of the hand by grasping a cardboard cone, either actively or passively. Each type of stimulation should be done for a minimum of two minutes though one can alternate 30 seconds rubbing and 30 seconds pressure. The patient should be told that the treatment should feel good and to tell the thrapist when he feels uncomfortable. Be on the alert for signs of discomfort, such as a slight withdrawal response when stroking the fingers. When evidence of discomfort is seen, change the stimulation to a new area to avoid activation of the protective response.

2. Vinograd, Taylor, and Grossman[227] reported a study in which patients improved on tests of stereognosis. The patients practiced discriminating different objects while manipulating them in an open end box whose bottom and three sides were mirrors. The patients practiced first with vision and then with vision occluded.

3. Believing that improvement in one task will transfer to similar tasks, have the patient practice, with vision occluded, discriminating different textures on a texture board, e.g., a piece of wood with various textures—sandpaper, silk, terrycloth—tacked on it.

Auditory Agnosia

Auditory agnosia is the inability to recognize differences in sounds, including both word and nonword sounds. For example, a patient may not be able to differentiate between the sound of a car engine running and the sound of a vacuum cleaner.

Lesion site: temporal lobe of the dominant hemisphere.[165]

Evaluation and Treatment of Auditory Agnosia

Evaluation and treatment for auditory agnosia are usually done by the speech therapist. However, if there is no speech therapist available, ask the patient to close his eyes and listen to different sounds and then identify their sources by pointing to them. For example, ring a bell and ask the patient to identify the source of the sound. Or ask the patient to point to body parts named to see whether he can differentiate between the sounds of different body parts. The examiner will probably have to use gestures to help the patient understand what he is being asked to do as verbal comprehension in these patients is usually limited.[223]

Treatment of this deficit is not very effective. Speech pathologists sometimes use retraining procedures such as drill in listening and making auditory discrimination and practice in discriminating visual forms, sizes, and colors. Some therapists believe that treatment is given more for the morale of the patient and his family than to provide actual benefit to him.

Apractognosia

Apractognosia consists of several different apraxic and agnostic syndromes, all centering mainly around a lack of perspective.*[122] Resulting from a lesion in the nondominant hemisphere, apractognosia may include one or all of the following:
1. Body scheme problems.
    a. Denial of left hemiplegia.
    b. Lack of awareness of left half of body or space.
    c. Feelings of strangeness.
    d. Right-left disorientation for both personal and extrapersonal space.
2. Apraxia for dressing.
    a. Faulty application of clothes to the body because the patient cannot understand the relationship of the clothes to the body.
    b. Faulty right-left manipulations used in tying a tie or a shoe.
3. Constructional apraxia due to lack of perspective.
4. Unilateral spatial agnosia.
    a. Loss of conception of topographical relationships such that the patient could no longer conceive that the bathroom is down the hall to the left of his room.
    b. Disturbances of orientation such that the patient does not know where he is.
    c. Loss of topographical memory such that the patient has forgotten his familiar routes from one place to another.

---

*This reference is a source of extensive information about apractognosia.

5. Visual coordinate problems such that the patient has difficulty perceiving the vertical and horizontal correctly.

Lesion site: parieto-occipital regions of the nondominant hemisphere.[122,165]

Evaluation and Treatment for Apractognosia

Evaluation and treatment for the apractognosia syndrome may be found under the corresponding apraxic and agnostic deficits on the following pages:

1. Body scheme disorders.
   a. Anosognosia, page 64.
   b. Unilateral neglect, page 59.
   c. Right-left disorientation, page 65.
2. Dressing apraxia, page 85.
3. Constructional apraxia for the nondominant hemisphere, page 84.
4. Visual spatial agnosia.
   a, b, and c. Topographical discrimination, page 85, and also under Spatial Relations Syndrome, page 81.

Agnosias Related to Body Scheme Disorders

Somatognosia: See this description under Body Image-Body Scheme Disorders, page 53.

Anosognosia: See this description under Body Image-Body Scheme Disorders, page 64.

CHAPTER VII

Factors That Complicate the Patient's Performance of Perceptual Tasks

Information about aphasia and sensory loss or disturbance (both cortical and peripheral) is included in this manual because these disorders may complicate or mask perceptual problems. In treating the hemiplegic patient, it is important first to evaluate both these areas before designing a program to improve perceptual function.

The authors have not included any evaluation or treatment for aphasia or sensory impairment as these are not basically perceptual problems. However, the therapist will want to coordinate treatment with the speech department for the aphasic patient. The reader is referred to Bobath[36] for treatment of sensory disturbance.

Aphasia and Dysphasia*

Aphasia can be classified into three major divisions[100]: expressive aphasia (also called verbal, motor, or Broca's aphasia), receptive aphasia (also called sensory, auditory, or Wernicke's aphasia), and conduction aphasia. Expressive aphasia, the inability to express oneself through speech although comprehension of spoken words is intact, is caused by a lesion in Broca's area, the anterior part of the association cortex located in the posterior inferior frontal gyrus.[100] Receptive aphasia, caused by a lesion in Wernicke's area, the temporoparietal area of the association cortex,[100] is the inability to comprehend the spoken word. Conduction aphasia, caused by a lesion in the arcuate fasciculus, an area between the brain locations for receptive and expressive aphasias,[100,125] results in intact comprehension of speech and expressive speech, although one is not able to bridge the two divisions. Thus, the patient would be unable to repeat sounds, as that would involve first perception and then related expression.[125]

It is believed that the language centers for 97 percent of the population occur in the left cerebral hemisphere.[128] More precisely, language centers for 99 percent of right-handed persons occur in the left hemisphere (60 percent for left-handed persons). Thus, for persons with lesions in the left cerebral hemisphere, some communication problems are highly likely. However, aphasia does infrequently occur following some right hemisphere lesions. For left-handed persons exhibiting aphasia after damage to the right hemisphere, studies have shown that they often have early histories of left hemisphere brain injury.[4] In right-handed persons with right hemisphere damage, studies have shown that the patient has problems related to the characteristics of speech, the language of voice and delivery, and a problem in language.[4]

Right hemisphere language problems are now being documented.

---

* The prefixes "a," meaning totally without, and "dys," meaning impairment of, are often used interchangeably when referring to these deficits.

Research indicates that key right hemisphere language difficulties include confusion, a decrease in processing and integrating information, decreased semantics, decreased verbal problem solving, and aprosadic speech.[54,127,209,217]

Because patients with aphasia are often confused and lack the ability to communicate, it is difficult to test them perceptually. Even tests that do not require verbal answers still require the patient first to understand verbal, written, or gestured instructions and then to formulate an answer that may involve language symbols in his silent mediation.[81] Timed tests also limit these patients. In a study by DeRenzi,[81] asphasics scored lowest on immediate memory tests in which, possibly, they did not have time to fully analyze questions and formulate mental answers. However, in memory tasks in which patients were given a longer time interval before answering, language difficulties were found to be significant.[81]

In further studies,[122,203,211] language and body scheme have been found to be closely related such that an intact body scheme may be dependent upon one's language facility. Sanguet, Benton, and Hecaen[203] suggest that receptive aphasia seems to be a prerequisite for significant defects in finger recognition and right-left discrimination. In another study by Hecaen et al.[122] it was hypothesized that the verbalization experience enters a sphere of concepts and symbols for which only the whole body has reality and is conceived as a point of reference to the outside world. Once a lesion occurs to upset his balance between language and body, the patient has lost his verbal body image and cannot name or point to the various parts of his body.[122,203,211]

The following symptoms are also part of the language disorder and are included in the glossary:
1. Receptive problems
    a. Alexia
    b. Asymbolia
2. Expressive problems
    a. Anomia
    b. Agrammatism
    c. Verbal apraxia
    d. Agraphia
    e. Acalculia
    f. Aphemia

Sensory Loss

Before doing perceptual testing or drawing conclusions about a patient's perceptual status, it is most important to know his level of remaining sensation. Diminished sensation complicates the evaluation of perceptual problems as it may be the cause of impaired motor planning, limb agnosia, and the inability to localize touch, pressure, and pain.[36] In a patient who no longer receives adequate limb sensation, motor planning for body parts becomes extremely difficult. Therefore, an incoordination or lack of execution that resembles an apraxia may, in fact, be caused by impaired sensation. Bobath[36] states that the influence of sensory loss may actually impair one's appreciation for size, shape, form, and textures and may possibly be the cause in some cases of tactile agnosia.

Vision

One of the primary mechanisms that shapes our perception is vision. Through underlying brain mechanisms, what we see is integrated and transformed into meaningful perceptions. The therapist must understand this relationship in order to accurately interpret the patient's performance in perceptual testing and during activities of daily living. In order for this relationship to be clearly understood, the therapist must have an understanding of vision and the visual process. A brief description of the visual process is presented and subsequently related to perception. For a detailed description of the visual system, the reader is referred to references 13, 62, and 196.

It is well known that every image we see has numerous edges and lines.[196] The eye absorbs light, and retinal cone cells distinguish different wavelengths and contrasts. In addition, there are some nerve cells that are sensitive to differences in tone or texture (for example, sunshine and water ripples).[196] Electrical images related to light, tone, texture, and the like leave the eye by the optic nerve and then travel toward the brain and specifically the visual cortex located in the occipital lobe. Behind the retina ". . . visual pathways in the two eyes cross with the inner fibers, passing to the opposite side."[196] The lens of the eye inverts the electrical and chemical signals, resulting in an upside down image, which is then encoded by brain mechanisms.

The encoding process of the impulses received by the eye involves the integration of many skeletal, visceral, cortical, and subcortical processes.[13,62] The specific functional visual components that assist in this integrative process are fixation, tracking, focusing and fusion.[62] The result of this integration by relevant brain functions is the brain's ability to understand what is seen according to size, shape, distance, and form. This understanding is perception.

Vision, then, extends beyond the basic sensory receptors for light and radiant energy. It involves an intricate process, which leads to the development of perception. When there is a breakdown at any point in the visual processing system, an associated perceptual loss will also occur.

The patient who has sustained a stroke may experience visual loss or

Figure 7-1. Visual deficits common to the brain damaged.

Deficit	Underlying Mechanism	Clinical Manifestation/Resulting Deficit	Treatment
Double vision	Decreased extraocular control preventing both eyes from seeing the same object simultaneously; for example, third nerve palsy (one eye will deviate)	In severe cases the brain will suppress one image and focus with one eye; in borderline cases (and with fatigue) the patient will actually see double	Eye patching (alternate eye patched at least once every one to two days)
Decreased convergence	Convergence-accommodation reflex: contraction of medial rectus muscles, lens thickening by ciliary muscles, narrowing of pupils	Double vision or blurred vision for close fields; decreased depth perception	Patient drills for convergence (i.e., object brought in toward patient's nose on which he must focus)
Blurred vision	Impaired innervation of the focusing muscles	Vision blurred for both close fields and for distance	Prescription lenses; not always correctable
Nystagmus	Brainstem damage (especially vestibular system); cerebellar damage	Abnormal oscillations of the eyes resulting in blurred vision (decreased visual acuity)	Surgery; sensory integration therapy (developed originally for use with learning disabled children but is being applied to the brain damaged adult)

Figure 7-1. Visual deficits common to the brain damaged (*continued*).

Deficit	Underlying Mechanism	Clinical Manifestation/ Resulting Deficit	Treatment
Visual field loss	Right or left temporal or parietal lobe; optic nerve, radiations or chiasmal lesion	A variety of field deficits depending on location of lesion; these can include scotomas, hemianopsias, and quadrantanopsias	Train the patient to compensate for the loss through effective visual scanning
Decreased oculomotor skills: 1. Ocular pursuits	Lesion in either hemisphere with or without brainstem damage	Difficulty or inability to track in any or all of the following planes, depending on location of damage: horizontal, oblique, vertical, or rotatory	Transfer of training approach; functional; computers and videogames; sensory motor approach
2. Saccadic eye movements	Frontal cortex (area 8)	Difficulty or inability in quick localization; difficulty with reading	Transfer of training; sensory motor approach; computers and videogames

impairment related either to age or brain damage related to the stroke itself. Age related changes can occur in the cornea, pupil, iris, lens, vitreous, and ciliary muscles of the eye.[133] These age related changes are described in detail in the section entitled "Relationship of Age to Perceptual and Cognitive Evaluation and Treatment" and therefore will not be covered in this section. Visual impairment related to the stroke itself can include visual field loss, decreased convergence, blurred vision, double vision, and nystagmus. The underlying mechanisms and clinical manifestation of these deficits are described in Figure 7-1. Any of the deficits described will result in ineffective processing of visual input, which in turn can result in perceptual disorders. Decreased convergence, for example, can result in decreased depth perception for close fields of vision. Blurred vision, which decreases the eye's ability to detect edges and lines, can result in poor form, size, and figure ground perception, to name a few.

The therapist must have a clear understanding of the patient's visual status prior to perceptual testing. Providing the patient with glasses when indicated can result in significant differences in patient performance. If there is a question of visual system impairment, the therapist should recommend that the patient be referred for an eye examination. In addition, the therapist should include as part of the perceptual evaluation an assessment of visual attention, oculomotor skills (pursuits and saccades), visual neglect, and visual fields. Once there is a clear picture of the patient's visual status, the therapist can more accurately interpret the results of the perceptual evaluation.

Before leaving this section, it is important to note that many occupational therapists are seeking additional optometric training and beginning to specialize in visual retraining. At the present time, patient caseloads include primarily children with developmental or sensory integrative disability that has affected their vision. There is promise, however, that the theory and techniques utilized with children may be effectively applied to adults. Some of these techniques are included in the treatment sections related to gross visual skills. It is important to note that some visual retraining activities should be performed only by a visual retraining specialist or optometrist. These activities would involve the use of prisms and other binocular instruments.

CHAPTER VIII

Cognitive Deficits

Cognition

In addition to more obvious sensory, motor, visual, and perceptual deficits, the patient who has sustained a stroke may have diminished cognitive abilities.[248] Cognitive processes include those of knowing and understanding, awareness, judgment, and decision making.[65] If an individual is unable to initiate, direct, and redirect mental activity, resultant behavioral deficits might include poor attention, memory, and learning, as well as incompleteness of thought and action. The individual's response may be stimulus bound[102] and stimulus dependent, and he may have difficulty in monitoring, inhibiting, and shifting his behavior.[159]

The task of identifying discrete cognitive processes for the purposes of clinical evaluation and treatment is difficult and their separation arbitrary. For instance, a patient with a memory problem will more than likely have additional deficits in mental flexibility and problem solving. Despite this difficulty in isolating specific cognitive deficits, several categories of impairment can be identified in the patient who has sustained a stroke and the severity of the problem evaluated. These categories, described in detail in this chapter, are attention, memory, initiation, judgment, insight, problem solving, abstraction, mental flexibility, and calculation ability.

Given these categories of dysfunction, the clinician is faced with the dilemma of measuring this dysfunction effectively. The clinical psychologist primarily utilizes psychometric testing for the evaluation of cognitive dysfunction. Psychiatrists utilize qualitative rating scales, whereas the neuropsychologist typically uses neuropsychodiagnostic testing. The occupational therapist, on the other hand, should measure the patient's cognitive deficits with a functional emphasis. Although it is not the occupational therapist's role to administer extensive psychometric testing, it is the therapist's role to evaluate the patient's "functional cognitive" deficits and develop a remediation plan. In addition, the therapist should be aware of the current cognitive evaluations being utilized by psychologists and other team members, in order to facilitate complete communication between team members and therefore improve the quality of the patient's overall treatment.

The evaluation sections of each cognitive category discussed in this chapter therefore contain descriptions of state of the art tests utilized primarily by psychologists as well as functional measures or structured clinical observations.

The format for each section, as in the visual and perceptual sections of the book, consists of the deficit description, associated lesion site, test descriptions, including scoring and level of standardization, and suggested treatment.

Attention

Attention is often used as a "catch all" term to describe many aspects of behavior. Attention is a function " . . . which ensures that cognitive processing is directed towards the significant features of the environment."[162] Attention is an active process that helps to determine which sensations and experiences are alerting and relevant to the individual. By deciding what we pay attention to, we decide what information is transferred from sensory memory to meaningful images that can be stored. Concentration deficits can prevent adequate attending, which in turn can affect memory. Effort and concentration are required for the processing of new information. "Attention is of short duration and variability, bringing rapidly altering data to the system for continual comparative assessment."[185]

There are two types of information processing that are related to attention — automatic and controlled processing. Controlled processing is utilized when new information is being considered. Automatic processing, on the other hand, occurs at a subcortical level.[242] Many clinicians are already aware of the behavior patients exhibit relative to these two types of processing. For example, the patient who has sustained a stroke requires conscious attention to complete even the simplest tasks.[242] Two disorders, focused attentional deficit and divided attentional deficit, are related to these processing concepts and can occur after a stroke. These terms are defined along with additional attention related terms at the end of this section.

Often the term attention is used interchangeably with other terms such as alertness, vigilance, or effort. This creates confusion and does not assist the therapist in identifying deficits and designing treatment programs. These terms therefore are defined in an effort to clarify related concepts, as follows:

Alertness. A component of attention. Alerting is more related to the periphery, preparing the individual to mobilize to attention, and theoretically functions through different neurological systems from attention;[43] a fluctuating condition of the central nervous system.[242]

Attention. A state of arousal allowing the individual to receive information and attend to it;[242] contains the three components of alertness, selectivity, and effort. Attention may be focused or divided and can vary in duration and intensity.[41,92]

Concentration-vigilance-effort. The ability to sustain attention over a period of time. Thirty seconds is considered a vigilant period in a mental status examination;[220] a control process that coordinates functional components of attention (alertness, arousal, and selectivity) to direct attention to significant features of the environment. Note: It is this aspect of attention that appears particularly vulnerable to brain damage.

Divided attention deficit. Occurs "when controlled processing is in use and where the limitations of the system fail to accommodate all the information necessary for optimal task performance."[242] This often results in patients becoming slow in processing and behavior and "overloaded" when they have to deal with several alternatives.

Focused attention deficit. Occurs "when an automatic response is replaced by a controlled response,"[242] for example, walking after a stroke.

Selective attention. The process of choosing some items of information rather than others; some items affect awareness, memory, and behavior more than nonselected items that may be present at the same time.[242]

Lesion site. Several areas have been implicated with attentional deficits:
   a. *Reticular activating system.* Arousal or alertness.[12,92,220]
   b. *Frontal and temporal lobes.* Direction of attention, intention to attend, concentration, and so forth.[92,152,162] Right hemispheric lesions appear to have a stronger effect than left sided lesions.[220]
   c. *Limbic system.* Associated with the emotional aspect of attention.[220]

Evaluation of Attention

Because memory, problem solving, and other higher intellectual functions all have an attentional component, attention should always be evaluated at the beginning of a functional cognitive evaluation.

TEST NO. 1: Random Letter Test[220]
Description: The evaluator reads a long list of random letters and asks the patient to somehow indicate (e.g., by nodding or tapping a finger) when he hears a predetermined letter. Letters are read at the rate of one per second.
Scoring: Nonstandardized. Patient should complete the task without any errors. Note any perseveration or omissions.
   To improve validity, rule out auditory or language deficits as causes of poor performance.

TEST NO. 2: Digit Repetition Test[220]
Description: The evaluator states random number sequences (starting with two and increasing until the patient fails) and asks the patient to say the same numbers after he or she is finished. Numbers are presented at the rate of one digit per second.
Scoring: Nonstandardized. A typical patient of average intelligence can repeat five to seven digits. Less than five indicates defective attention.
   To improve validity, rule out auditory or language deficits as causes of poor performance.

TEST NO. 3: Clinical Observation and Activity Analysis
General Guidelines for Evaluation
   1. Identify the components of attention (e.g., alerting, selectivity, effort) that are intact and those that are impaired.

2. Observe the patient in a number of settings and activities at different times during the day. Position change (lying, sitting) can also affect attention.
3. Establish functional baseline measures. Consider the frequency and severity of the problem. Select relevant functional tasks as the basis for the evaluation and reassessment.

Specific Areas or Questions to Consider and Evaluate

1. Which sensory systems are affected? Visual? Auditory?
2. What are the duration and frequency of the patient's attentional abilities?
3. Under what environmental conditions can the patient attend to a task? When does attention begin to break down?
4. What are some behavioral indications of the patient's inattention?
5. Does the patient have memory problems? Does he have problem solving difficulties? Decreased processing? Are these or related problems caused in part by decreased attention?
6. Are there any tasks or areas that seem to particularly interest the patient and therefore increase his attention?
7. Is processing occurring only at a conscious level as opposed to a normal combination of automatic and conscious?

Scoring: Nonstandardized. The foregoing and similar questions can be incorporated into a checklist or used in conjunction with a frequency rating scale (e.g., always/sometimes/rarely/never).

To improve validity, rule out auditory and language problems as the causes of poor performance.

Treatment of Attention Deficits

1. Applying the concept that environment can affect performance:
   a. Begin training in a nondistracting environment with structure as needed. As the patient improves, progress to a more normal environment and gradually lessen the structure required.
   b. Note changes in observable behavior in all environments and functions related to attention to a task. Provide external feedback to modify behavior as needed. Reward the patient in proportion to the length of time he attends to the task.[242]
   c. Increase the time and duration of treatment as well as the complexity of the task as the patient improves.
   d. Provide appropriate external cuing. For example, teach the patient to screen out distractions and use environmental cues to determine the most appropriate response.[187] Also teach the patient to actively scan his environment, seek out the presence of cues, and identify them.[187,194]

e. Assist the patient in developing and utilizing internal attentional strategies, such as the following:

   i. The patient could be taught statements to prepare himself to listen and ask for repetition if his attention strays,[233] e.g., "I must really concentrate and look at the person speaking to me."

   ii. Have the patient vocalize step by step as he performs a task. Progress to subvocalization (patient silently vocalizes), thereby internalizing the technique.[233]

   f. Help the patient with the attentional components of a task before having him develop cognitive strategies related to the task.[242] In other words, treat the attentional deficit first.

2. In an attempt to utilize sensory input (visual, tactile, auditory) in relation to motor output (e.g., attention to task, participation in task), provide controlled sensory cuing with the patient subsequently demonstrating active interaction with the environment. Initially provide sensory cuing separately, for example, visual, auditory or tactile. Once the patient is able to respond to single system cues, provide multisystem cues.[86]

3. Assuming that improvement in one task will transfer into another, have the patient engage in activities such as maze learning or serial memory skills. An example of transfer of training activity would be to provide the patient with a random number chart with the numbers written in different colors. Have the patient call out the colors that the numbers are on.[67]

4. Some clinicians advocate the use of videogames and computers for the remediation of attentional deficits.[213]

5. Utilizing a multimodality approach, apply several of the treatment strategies described.

Memory

Memory is not a single factor but one that relates to learning and perception.[170] One must attend to and perceive something before it can be remembered. Memory is essentially perception that has been stored at an earlier time and then can be brought forward.[43] It can exist across all sensory modalities or be modality specific, and any sense or combination of senses can elicit a recollection.[58,143] It is a dynamic process involving many associated components.

No matter what definition one utilizes for memory, the underlying concept that it includes permanent change in the central nervous sytem, which can later be reproduced, appears to be universally accepted.[92] The constant interaction between an individual and the environment elicits memories, which can be retrieved in an exact or equivalent form.[92] Memory requires input from the environment (both internal and external), change within the the central nervous system, maintenance of that change, and an output (behavioral or informational) that somehow consistently relates to the input.[92]

The memory process begins with the input of sensations. The individual selectively attends to the environment, depending on his interests at the time of a given sensory input from the environment. The input is placed in sensory memory and changed into images, which then travel to the sensory areas of the brain.[92]

The process continues from sensory memory to short term memory, which is considered to be a temporary storage. This temporary storage acts as part of a control mechanism for higher intellectual processing and functions.[92] From short term memory, items are encoded and consolidated into long term memory. New information must be organized and categorized with what has already been learned. Memory may be organized or classified as semantic memory (memory for knowledge) or episodic memory.[16] Examples of episodic memory are remembering what one has had for breakfast or when the next holiday is. The consolidation process of this stage takes minutes or hours and can be stored in long term memory — in some cases for a lifetime.[16,92,152]

Retrieval of stored information is the final aspect of the memory process. Short term memory selects an access code that will retrieve information with a similar code.[92] The information is subsequently moved from long to short term memory.[92] Retrieval, then, is the process of locating and removing items from long term memory storage. It is an active process of mobilizing stored items.[220]

Before evaluating and treating memory disorders, a clear understanding of related terms and concepts is crucial. Figure 8-1 defines relevant terms pertaining to memory and associated lesion sites for specific memory deficits.

Evaluation of Memory

Memory assessment should be considered in conjunction with many other cognitive functions. Consideration should be given to speed, attention, reasoning, and the ability to inhibit responses.[46] Many materials have been used to evaluate memory, but there has been little standardization of the tests utilized.[119] Additional problems exist even in standardized tests. Many do not specify the particular problems, or the frequency or severity of the problems, as related to memory deficit.[239] Many are not relevant to activities of daily living, and this may cause problems in motivation.[239] Self-report (or family report) memory scales purport to answer to some of these problems.[239] The major problem with these scales is biases, which influence accuracy and validity.[26]

As noted earlier, the occupational therapist's role in cognitive evaluation and treatment should emphasize function. It is important, however, that the therapist be aware of the measures being utilized by other members of the treatment team. With this in mind, a description of the most commonly used standardized memory test and an example of a self-report memory questionnaire are provided. The remaining information (listed under Test No. 3) covers guidelines for structured observation and activity analysis as related to memory and function.

TEST NO. 1: Wechsler Memory Scale[234]

Description: Subtests include Personal and Current Information, Orientation, Mental Control, Logical Memory, Digit Span, Visual Reproduction, and Associative Learning.

Scoring: The Wechsler Memory Scale tests four types of memory: short term memory digit span, associative verbal memory, meaningful verbal memory, and figural memory.[92]

To improve validity, rule out visual, perceptual, language, and attentional deficits as causes of poor performance.

Reliability: Norms by Wechsler are available to age 64.[234,235]

TEST NO. 2: The Subjective Memory Questionnaire[26]

Description: This scale consists of 43 items relating to everyday life. These items cover areas such as people's names, facts about people, film titles, jokes, and directions to get somewhere.

Scoring: Two different 5-point rating scales are utilized. The first 36 items are answered on a "very good" to "very bad" scale. Items 37 to 43 are temporal and are answered on a "very rarely" to "very often" scale.

To improve validity, rule out attentional and language related problems as causes of poor performance.

Reliability: Test-retest reliability has been established ($p<0.001$) on this questionnaire.[26] Item correlations also indicated "high positive item to test correlations."[26]

TEST NO. 3: Clinical Observation and Activity Analysis

General Guidelines for Evaluation

1. Identify the aspects of memory that are impaired and those that are relatively intact.

Figure 8-1. Memory (Types, Description, and Associated Lesion Site)[44,63,92,146,152,157,198,220]

Types and Components of Memory	Definition and Description	Associated Lesion Site
1. Recognition	A factor inherent in recall; a primitive memory function that serves to alert one to the surroundings by focusing and shifting attention	Thalamus
2. Iconic	Sensory memory; the initial processing of the information after the input sensation has been received by sense organs	Predominantly a retinal phenomenon mediated by rod vision
3. Short term (also called immediate, primary span, short term store, recent)	Length is only 20 to 40 seconds; 5 to 10 items can be held in short term memory; retention span of events, objects, or ideas in immediate awareness; constitutes consciousness, since people are aware of cognitive processes that are not automatic	Fontal lobe: Verbal—left hemisphere Nonverbal—right hemisphere
4. Long term (also called secondary, delayed, distant, remote)	Represents permanent record of learned material; has three stages—consolidation, storage, and retrieval of stored memory	

Figure 8-1. Memory *(continued)*

Types and Components of Memory	Definition and Description	Associated Lesion Site
a. Consolidation	Involves transfer of material into long term memory and its consolidation; strengthens memory trace to facilitate permanence; material is coded during the transfer process	Hippocampus: Verbal—left hippocampus Nonverbal—right hippocampus Limbic system (thalamus, mammillary bodies, fornix)
b. Storage	Relatively permanent storage of materials that have been consolidated; two categories of long term memory storage are: 1. Episodic—information related to events with temporal and spatial components (when and where) 2. Semantic—memory with no temporal or spatial content (e.g, words, symbols)	Lateral surface of temporal lobe Anterior portion of right or left temporal lobe
c. Retrieval (recall)	Higher level cognitive function is dependent upon lower functioning recognition; permits creativity and planning; takes two forms—direct verbatim access or access to a general idea of the original material; successful retrieval requires the availability of information in storage and access to that information at the desired time	Temporal lobe Hippocampus Thalamus

2. Observe the patient in a number of settings.
3. Consider the amount of structure versus nonstructure within the environment.
4. Consider the time interval between stimulus and recall (i.e., immediate, short term, and long term).
5. Establish functional baseline measures. Consider the frequency and severity of the problem as it relates to function. Select relevant functional areas or tasks as the basis for evaluation and reassessment.

Specific Areas and Questions to Consider and Evaluate

1. Which sensory system is affected? For instance, immediate recall can be tested for different sensory systems as follows:[58,228,247]
   a. *Visual*. The patient is asked to reproduce simple geometric figures, which are presented for 5 to 10 seconds and then covered.[58,228,247] Note: If a person's perceptual abilities are impaired, it is likely that this will affect memory for visual material and the ability to use visually based strategies to assist in memory problems.[46]
   b. *Kinesthetic*. The patient is asked to reproduce a series of hand positions presented to him.[58]
   c. *Auditory*. The patient is asked to reproduce a series of rhythmic taps.[58] Note: If the patient is aphasic, verbal memory and the ability to use verbal memory strategies are likely to be affected.
2. Is nonverbal memory impaired? Verbal memory?
3. Is memory loss global or modality specific?
4. Is it a learning or a performance problem? Can the patient improve with practice?
5. Is it a problem of learning new information or recalling old information?
6. Which memory processes are affected? Does the patient have trouble identifying as well as reproducing (recall versus recognition)?
7. Is it a semantic memory loss? Is it episodic?
8. Does the patient have difficulty with free recall?
9. Does the patient have difficulty with serial learning (i.e., remembering sequences)?
10. Does the patient have difficulty with paired associates (i.e., remembering relationships)?

Scoring: Nonstandardized. The foregoing or similar questions can be incorporated into a checklist (yes/no) or used in conjunction with a frequency rating scale (example: always/sometimes/rarely/never). To improve validity, rule out perceptual, language, and attentional deficits as causes of poor performance.

Treatment of Memory Deficits

Applying the concept that environment can affect performance:

a. Maintain a consistent repetitive routine and environment from day to day.

b. Control the amount and duration of external structure and adaptations provided within the environment. A little memory training provided more often has been found to be more effective than too much for too long.[16] For example, in learning someone's name, ". . . if you present this information twice, the presenting it twice in quick succession leads to less learning than presenting it twice with a few minutes delay. . ."[16] Minimize the structure and adaptations provided as the patient improves.

c. Assist the patient in developing and effectively utilizing both internal and external environmental memory aids and strategies. Teaching memory strategies rather than repetitive drills may help the patient generalize to everyday learning.[198] Teach the patient organizational and encoding skills.[182]

The following are examples of internal and external memory aids, and organizational and encoding strategies.

Internal Aids. *Rehearsal.*[9,92,104] The patient repeats silently or out loud information to be retained. Repeating an item will increase the time of attention paid to that item and so reinforces its memory.[92] Rehearsal maintains items in short term memory, codes them, and transfers them into long term memory.[9,92]

Elaborating. The patient works on the detail of the information and relates it to what he already knows.[143,160]

Compatibility. The patient forms a judgment that the information is consistent with what he already knows.[143]

Self-reference. The patient judges how the material relates to him. This has been found to assist retention more than relating it to others.[143]

Visual Imagery. The patient forms a visual image in his mind related to the information to be recalled.[57,73,145,174]

Mnemonics. One or more of the following can be utilized:[24,64,118,160,182,174]

a. First letter mnemonics. The first letters of the words within a phrase represent the first letters of the words or information to be recalled.[233] Many occupational therapists utilize this method to memorize the cranial nerves: e.g., "Old obstetricians often try to abduct fair and glamorous virgins somehow."[233]

b. Pegword mnemonics. A peg word is used to cue the patient to various tasks, e.g.:

      S - shopping

      L - laundry

      E - eat lunch

      E - exercise

      P - pick up children at school [118]

c. Rhyming mnemonics. A word that rhymes with the word or information to be recalled is utilized, e.g., fun-sun, heaven-seven.

d. P.Q.R.S.T. method[104]

    1. Preview. The patient skims the material to learn the general content.

    2. Question. The patient asks himself key questions about the content.

    3. Read. The patient reads the information with the goal of answering the question.

    4. State. The patient repeats or rehearses the information read.

    5. Test. The patient tests himself by answering the questions he posed previously.

e. Story method. The patient forms a story about the words or phrases he is to remember.[102]

External Aids. General principles of effective external cuing include the following:[118]

1. Give the cuing as close as possible to the time the action is required.

2. Make it active.

3. Be specific about what is required.

4. If using a device:

    a. Make it portable. The device should be able to store as many cues as possible.

    b. It should have as wide a time range as possible.

    c. It should be easy to use and not be dependent on any other instrument.

Specific types of external cues include the following:

1. Use of timetables, diaries, tests, pictures, plans, and written instructions.

2. Alarm clocks, watch alarms, and various electronic memory aids.

3. The use of chaining — breaking down the task into steps (links) and teaching one step at a time. Once one step is learned, another is added and then another, and so on.[239]

4. Adapting the external environment, e.g., labeling doors and color coding.

5. Providing verbal or visual retrieval cues. This will encourage a focused search in memory.[72] Questioning the patient during presenta-

tion appears to assist in retention.[71] Retrieval cues that are similar to those used in the original learning process can be especially helpful to recall.[46]

Note: It is hoped, and has been observed in some cases, that repetitive use of external cuing will eventually lead the patient to utilize the cues internally. For example, verbal questioning (as described in item 5 above) should also help teach the patient how to ask the questions that will help his memory. Once a skill has been achieved or remembered, have the patient practice it in as wide a range of environments as possible.[16]

1. In an attempt to utilize sensory input (visual, kinesthetic, verbal memory) in relation to a motor output (recall), utilize the remaining intact sensory systems in treatment. For example, use visual imagery (internal) or pictures (external) if the patient has poor auditory or verbal skills. Conversely, use verbal cuing with the patient whose visual system is affected.[16,31,40]

2. Assuming that improvement in one task will transfer over into another, have the patient engage in puzzles, memory games, card games (concentration), and video games.

3. Some clinicians advocate the use of video games and computers for memory retraining.

4. Utilizing a multimodality approach, apply several of the treatment strategies described.

Note: In memory retraining always determine which deficits are responding to treatment and which improve with practice. Always keep post-therapy goals in mind and keep them realistic and functional.

Initiation

Difficulty in initiating or starting a task may be revealed by decreased spontaneity, decreased productivity, slowness of response, or absence of initiative.[147] The patient with an initiation problem may be able to plan, organize, and carry out complex tasks, but only when instructed to do so.[147] The patient with a bilateral lesion may also demonstrate indifference, apathy, and general lethargy.[162] Depending on the exact lesion site, the patient may also have difficulty with the control, regulation, processing, and integration of cognitive tasks.[147]

Lesion site: frontal lobe.

Evaluation of Initiation

TEST NO. 1: Clinical Observation and Activity Analysis
General Guidelines for Evaluation
1. Observe the patient in a number of settings.

2. Consider the amount of structure and cuing required for initiation of activity by the patient.
3. Establish functional baseline measures. Consider the frequency and severity of the problem as it relates to function. Select relevant functional areas or tasks as the basis for evaluation and reassessment.

Specific Areas and Questions to Consider and Evaluate

1. Are there any associated behavioral problems, such as flat or blunted affect? Behavioral outbursts? Disinhibition?
2. Is the patient's behavior generally passive? Does he respond passively to questions or suggestions?
3. What does the patient do during the day? Does someone have to organize his activity for him?
4. What, if any, activities can the patient initiate by himself without cuing or structure?
5. What cuing method or sensory modality appears to be the most effective? For example, do tactile or kinesthetic cues work better than visual or auditory cues?
6. Is the patient aware that he has an initiation problem? Does he accept it when it is pointed out to him?
7. Is an associated attentional or memory problem affecting initiation abilities?

To improve validity, rule out decreased attention, processing, language, apraxia, and psychologically based (versus organic) depression as causes of poor performance.

Treatment of Initiation Deficits

1. Applying the concept that environment can affect performance:
   a. Provide external cuing to assist the patient in initiating selected tasks. Control the amount and duration of cuing provided. Decrease the cuing as the patient's initiation skills improve.
   b. Assist the patient in developing an awareness of the problem so that he can begin to develop his own internal cuing system for initiating tasks.
2. In an attempt to utilize sensory input (visual, auditory, kinesthetic, and tactile) in relation to motor output (initiation), provide controlled sensory stimulation in treatments. For example, tactile and kinesthetic stimulation of the patient's arm combined with auditory cuing may be utilized to cue the patient to initiate upper extremity dressing.

Planning and Organization

The ability to learn and achieve any goal necessitates organization and planning. In order to formulate a goal, the individual must be able to determine what he needs and wants, and foresee the future realization of these needs.[116,146] The determination and organization of the steps needed to achieve a goal involve several component skills of planning. In order to plan, the individual must be able to conceptualize change from the present situation, relate objectively to the environment, conceive alternatives, weigh alternatives and make a choice, and develop a structure or framework to give direction to the carrying out of the plan.[147]

The patient who has sustained a stroke can have difficulty with planning and goal attainment. He may in fact lack the foresight and sustained attention necessary for achieving a desired goal. Often the patient can describe in detail the elements in planning and organizing impersonal events, but shows poor, unrealistic, or illogical plans for himself.[147] There may be varying degrees of planning and organizational deficits in such patients.[66]

Lesion site: frontal lobes.[66,92,147]

Evaluation of Planning and Organization

TEST NO. 1: Clinical Observation and Activity Analysis
General Guidelines for Evaluation
1. Determine whether the patient is aware that he has a planning deficit. Defective planning often can be revealed by asking the patient what he intends to do.
2. Observe the patient in a number of settings and activities during the day. Can the patient plan for activities requiring two step operations? Three step? More complex operations?
3. Establish functional baseline measures. Consider the duration and frequency of the problem. Select relevant functional tasks as the basis of evaluation and reassessment.

Specific Areas and Questions to Consider and Evaluate[67,194]

1. Is the patient logical and consistent in his approach to the task?
2. How reliable is his chosen method?
3. Is there a common problem or consistent faulty planning strategy that is generalized to several activities?
4. Can the patient conceptualize change (as evidenced through verbal or other means of communication) from the present?
5. Can the patient present alternatives to an established plan?
6. Can he weigh these alternatives and make a choice based on his judgments?
7. Does he appear to have a framework for the plan or direction he is demonstrating for task completion?

Note: Questions and observations such as these can be applied to both functional and cognitive perceptual motor tasks. For example, inability to complete block designs (refer to Test No. 1 in the problem solving section) and layout of graphic designs can be indicative of poor planning and task organization.

Scoring: Nonstandardized. These and similar questions can be incorporated into a checklist or used in conjunction with a frequency rating scale (e.g., always/sometimes/rarely/never).

To improve validity, rule out decreased attention, poor memory, impaired problem solving, and aphasia as causes of poor performance.

Treatment of Planning and Organization Deficits

1. Applying the concept that environment can affect performance:
   a. Control the amount and duration of feedback and structure provided within the environment.
   b. Assist the patient in developing and effectively utilizing both internal and external environmental planning aids. A sample external planning aid might include written, visual, or verbal step by step instructions for task completion. Internal environmental planning would involve verbal (out loud progressing to silent or internal) questioning by the patient.

   Self-questioning techniques might progress as follows:

   - What is it I want to accomplish?
   - What changes need to occur to move from the present situation to my desired goal?
   - What are the possible ways to make the necessary changes?
   - What is the sequence or order of steps required to make the changes?
   - Are there any alternatives to my plan? Which is the best alternative to use to reach my goal?
   - How will I know that I have reached my goal and that my plan was successful?

   As the patient asks these questions of himself, he can jot down his ideas or thought processes as an additional cuing mechanism. Analysis of this written plan by the therapist can then be utilized to identify any faulty planning or judgments. The patient then is encouraged to develop alternative strategies.

2. In the belief that improvement in one task will transfer over

124

into another, have the patient engage in puzzles, constructional tasks, and other relevant table top activities that require planning for task completion.
3. Utilizing a functional approach, have the patient plan and cook a meal or plan a community trip.
4. Utilizing a multimodality approach, apply several of the treatment strategies described.

Mental Flexibility and Abstraction

Many patients who have sustained a stroke have difficulty in conceptual thinking. A concrete attitude is common in which experiences, objects, and behavior are all interpreted by the patient at the most obvious, concrete value.[147] Some researchers consider memory deficits as a partial cause of concrete thinking.[31,170] Severe anterograde amnesia in cases of head injury is associated with subtle or severe problems with abstraction and decreased "mental flexibility," which in turn results in the patient's inability to learn and integrate new information for future conceptualization.[31] Theoretically, patients with poor abstraction and decreased mental flexibility are unable to perceive similarities and differences or to identify the important features in objects and events, because they are unable to keep these objects and events in mind.[170] Owing to a memory deficit, they are unable to make comparisons or are unable to retain the comparisons they have already made.

Decreased mental flexibility is often manifested by perseverative behavior. The patient may work with an idea and, if unsuccessful with this idea, be unable to generate new ideas.[66] The patient may show poor association ability and have difficulty in evaluating the relevance of the result obtained for a given problem.[58] This stimulus-bound or perseverative behavior makes it difficult for the patient to generalize knowledge for future problem solution.

Lesion site: frontal lobe.

Evaluation of Mental Flexibility

TEST NO. 1: Odd-Even Cross-out[66]

Description: This task tests the patient's ability to shift from one task to another. The patient is provided with a visual search worksheet with a series of numbers on it. He is asked to begin crossing out all the even numbers, and partially through the task is asked to cross out only the odd numbers. This instruction is subsequently reversed back to the even numbers, then back to the odd, and so on.

Scoring: Nonstandardized.

Intact: The patient is able to shift back and forth (odd-even) on all occasions as requested by the therapist.

Impaired: The patient is able to shift back and forth (odd-even) for only a portion of the task.

Unable: The patient is unable to successfully make the switch.

To improve validity, rule out decreased attention, decreased comprehension, visual neglect, visual field deficits, and decreased visual scanning as causes of poor performance.

Evaluation of Abstraction

TEST NO. 1: Concept Formation and Abstraction[58]

Concept formation involves the ability to define objects, compare and differentiate, establish logical relationships, and categorize. The following sample questions illustrate the evaluation of each of these components of concept formation and abstraction.[58]

1. Definition-abstraction. The patient is asked to define a specific word, e.g., chair, apple.

Scoring: Nonstandardized. The therapist notes how the patient makes use of abstract categories.

2. Comparison-differentiation. The patient is asked to relate a pair of ideas through:
   a. Common ground, e.g., refrigerator and stove, dresser and sofa.
   b. Differences, e.g., the difference between a fox and a dog, or a bed and a chair.

Scoring: Nonstandardized. The therapist notes whether the patient is able to identify similarities and differences between the paired ideas presented.

3. Logical relationships. The patient is asked to relate a word to a given series, e.g., a dog is an ——————, a knife is a ——————.

Scoring: Nonstandardized. The therapist notes the patient's ability to establish logical relationships through completion of the series presented.

4. Opposites. The patient is asked to supply the opposite of the word the therapist gives him, e.g., high-low, tall-short.

Scoring: Nonstandardized. The therapist notes the patient's ability to supply the opposite.

5. Categories. The patient is asked to identify the word that does not belong in a series of words the therapist provides, e.g., father, mother, brother, sister, friend.

Scoring: Nonstandardized. The therapist notes the patient's ability to identify the word that does not belong in the series.

To improve validity, rule out decreased attention, memory, and aphasia (especially comprehension) as causes of poor performance.

TEST NO. 2: Proverbs[220]

Description: The patient is asked to give the meaning of a series of proverbs supplied by the therapist; e.g., Rome wasn't built in a day; a stitch in time saves nine.

Scoring: Nonstandardized.

Intact: Abstract response.

Impaired: Semiabstract response.

Severely impaired: Concrete response.

To improve validity, rule out decreased attention, memory, and aphasia as causes of poor performance.

Treatment for Mental Flexibility

1. Utilizing a functional approach, ask the patient to perform, for example, a kitchen task that includes hot and cold meal preparation and functional categorization. Observe whether the patient can shift and organize his behavior within the overall activity.
2. Assuming that improvement in one task will aid improvement in another, have the patient perform table top activities that require numerous mental shifts and variations within the task, e.g., tasks involving shifting from color to the written word, or the substitution of visual instructions for verbal instructions.
3. Some clinicians advocate the use of computers in the remediation of mental flexibility.
4. Utilizing a multimodality approach, apply several of the treatment strategies described.

Decreased Insight and Impulsivity

The patient who has sustained a stroke often has poor awareness or insight into the limitations associated with his disorder. A patient may be totally unaware of blatant deficits that are obvious to those around him.[92] Some patients deny that they have a problem, to the point of becoming hostile to those who attempt to point deficits out. Still others may be indifferent to their limitations. Other patients may exhibit complete denial and resort to fabrication when someone is pointing out a deficit area.[220]

The patient's decreased insight into his disability will result in aberrant behavior, such as impulsiveness and poor safety awareness. He will be unable to correct any errors or mistakes because he is unable to perceive them.[147] Some patients may be able to perceive their errors but are unable to correct them. In general, the patient with poor insight is unable to monitor, self-correct, and regulate the quality of his behavior and performance. This inability to control and monitor his behavior will in turn affect his judgment in all functional tasks. The patient, for example, may impulsively try to get out of bed and walk to the bathroom in spite of his paralysis. Or he may be unsafe around the stove because of poor insight.

Lesion site: nondominant hemisphere, frontal lobe.[66,147,220]

Evaluation of Decreased Insight

TEST NO. 1: Clinical Observation and Activity Analysis

General Guidelines for Evaluation

1. Determine whether the patient is aware of and responsive to his environment. One measure of the patient's awareness is his ability to utilize feedback.[147]
2. Observe the patient in a number of settings and activities during the day. His limited insight, poor safety awareness, and impulsiveness can vary depending on the setting and the task.
3. Establish functional baseline measures. Consider the degree and frequency of the problem. Select relevant functional tasks as the basis of evaluation and reassessment.

Specific Areas and Questions to Consider and Evaluate

1. Can the patient perceive and verbalize (or somehow communicate) the extent and type of problems he is having?
2. Is he willing to try to understand and accept his problems when they are pointed out to him?
3. Once he admits that he has a specific problem, can he then perceive how it will affect his overall function beyond a specific task?
4. How does the environment affect the patient's awareness and behavior? Does a quiet structured environment decrease impulsivity and increase insight? In which environments does safety become an issue, e.g., kitchen, community?
5. Does verbal, visual, or tactile cuing improve insight or decrease impulsiveness?
6. What are the duration and frequency of the patient's impulsiveness and decreased insight or safety awareness?
7. Is there a task or tasks that are particularly helpful in illustrating a specific problem to the patient?

Scoring: Nonstandardized.

These and similar questions can be incorporated into a checklist or used in conjunction with a frequency rating scale (e.g., always/sometimes/rarely/never).

To improve validity, rule out decreased attention, poor memory, and aphasia as causes of poor performance.

Treatment of Decreased Insight

1. Applying the concept that environment can affect performance
   a. Treat the patient in a nondistracting environment as needed.
   b. Provide close monitoring and feedback. Feedback should

include discussion, observation, demonstration, and repetition as needed.[66]

c. Provide tasks that will gradually point out deficits. Although honesty is the best approach, this must be provided in conjunction with continued patient support. The therapist must not only point out patient limitations, but must concurrently point out strengths as well. The object of increasing the patient's insight is to facilitate safety and increase function, not to overwhelm the patient and create long term depression. Some initial depression will occur as the patient faces up to his limitations; however, if this depression persists, a referral to a psychologist may be indicated.

2. In an attempt to utilize sensory input (visual, auditory and tactile) in relation to motor output (decreased impulsiveness), provide controlled sensory cuing, with the patient subsequently demonstrating appropriate behavior during the desired activity.

a. For example, verbal and tactile cuing can be used prior to a kitchen task to increase the patient's safety awareness relative to his paralysis and sensory loss.

b. Videotaping the patient during treatment can be an effective visual cuing tool to increase the patient's insight into his disability. The tape should be played back at the end of the treatment session, with discussion pertaining to impulsive behavior or poor insight. The therapist must be honest yet supportive in the discussion of the patient's performance.

Problem Solving

Problem solving is not a single function, but rather the integration of several cognitive skills. Implicit in problem solving are attention to task, information access (both sensory from the environment and memory), organization, planning, and judgment.[41,58,185] Problem solving can vary depending, for instance, on whether the patient has access to and utilizes a memory aid.[41] Approaching a problem and comparing past and present experiences through memory skills enable an individual to think in an orderly manner.[170,193] The individual must be able to screen out and discard irrelevant information.[129,144,206] Once the information is registered and screened, the individual must be able to modify, transform, and organize it to come up with a solution.[41,58] Finally, the individual must be able to make judgments about the quality of potential solutions.[41]

Ben-Yishay et al.[31] summarized well the process of problem solving in 10 steps:

1. Begin with a problem.
2. Formulate it in an active and dynamic cognitive act by the person within the particular context in which it occurs.
3. An analysis must be undertaken of the conditions of this problem that are the most pertinent — in the given context — to a solution.
4. When the analysis is completed and the salient features of the problem have been identified by the person, the next phase in the process begins — choosing a strategy of approach to the solution from presenting alternatives.
5. Once a strategy of approach has been decided upon, the person must commence the task of formulating a working plan, which involves the setting of priorities, the formulation of operationalized action sequences, the determination of specific tactics to be employed, and the careful correlating of these so that they make up a coherent and continuous working plan.
6. Following the completion of this process, the person enters into the phase of executing the plan.
7. This in turn requires constant self-monitoring (of one's behavior) and the verification of the fact that each action sequence is being executed according to the original plan of action.
8. If all goes well, the person then arrives at a solution to the problem.
9. He must then compare the solution obtained with the original problem.
10. Once the solution is found to be acceptable, the person will perform an (explicit or implicit) mental act of evaluating the meaning and the significance of the given achievement. This cognitive process will culminate in the integration of the particular achievement just attained and with the person's other relevant goals and behaviors.[31]

In the patient who has sustained a stroke, the inability to solve problems may be due in part to an inability to process complex information, which can result in the patient's developing inappropriate strategies for solving given problems.[37] As a result, the patient may think concretely or appear to be impulsive. Another potential cause of such a patient's poor ability to solve problems is an inability to establish appropriate organizational strategies.[193] Some researchers believe that the difficulty is not in processing or developing appropriate strategies but rather the inadequate evaluation of these strategies and potential solutions.[41] It is more than likely that the patient who has sustained a stroke can have difficulty in any or all of these aspects of problem solving. An evaluation of problem solving, therefore, should incorporate as many components of problem solving as possible.

Lesion site: frontal lobe.

Evaluation of Problem Solving

TEST NO. 1: Cognitive Strategies — Block Design[247]

Description: The patient is asked to reproduce a block design that the examiner has constructed. While the patient is performing the task, the evaluator records his progression of attempts on the cognitive strategies worksheet (Figure 8-2).*

Scoring: Nonstandardized.

Intact: The patient approaches the problem in a meaningful organized way and evaluates his solution in comparison with the stimulus.

Impaired: The patient's approach is disorganized (trial and error); he or she is unable to make comparisons and judgments about the solution and the stimulus.

To improve validity, rule out spatial aspect constructional apraxia as a cause of poor performance. Note: the examiner is focusing not on whether the patient can complete the task, but rather on how he or she completes it or attempts to complete it.

TEST NO. 2: Clinical Observations and Activity Analysis[41],†

Description: Problem solving is divided into three stages: preparation, production, and judgment. Clinical observations in selected activities are based on questions related to these three stages as follows:

1. Preparation and understanding the problem (problem analysis)
   a. Can the patient identify any or all elements of the problem?
   b. Can the patient identify solution criteria?
   c. Can the patient identify any limitations or constraints related to potential attempts at problem solving?
   d. Can he describe or indicate how the problem compares with those he's already solved?
   e. Can the patient divide the problem into parts or components?
   f. Can the patient construct a simpler problem by ignoring some information?
2. Production: generating possible solutions
   a. Can the patient retrieve necessary information from long term memory?
   b. Can or does the patient scan the environment for available information?
   c. Can or does the patient operate or act on the content in short term memory?
   d. Can or does the patient store information in long term memory for later use?
   e. Can the patient generate a potential solution?

---

* Cognitive strategies worksheet adapted and reproduced with permission from Santa Clara Valley Medical Center, San Jose, California.

† Adapted and reproduced with permission from Prentice-Hall, Inc., Englewood Cliffs, New Jersey.

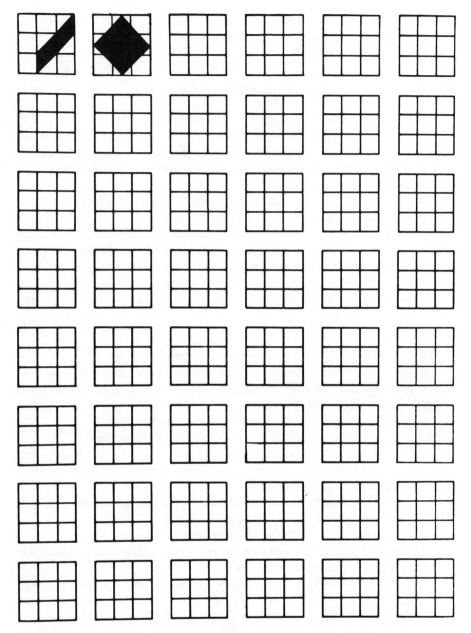

Figure 8-2. Cognitive strategies worksheet.

132

3. Judgment: evaluating the solutions generated
   a. Does the patient compare the generated solution with the initial solution criteria?
   b. Does the patient decide either that the problem has been solved or that more work is needed?

Scoring: Nonstandardized. The preceding or similar questions can be incorporated into a yes/no checklist or related to a frequency rating scale.

To improve validity, rule out poor attention, memory, impulsiveness, or other factors as causes of poor performance.

Treatment of Problem Solving Deficits

1. Applying the concept that environment can affect performance:
   a. Monitor how the task or environment can be altered in order to improve problem solving skills.
   b. Provide external cues to reduce the patient's use of inappropriate strategies.[37]
   c. Instruct the patient to check for errors before proceeding.
   d. When giving external cues, remember that you know how to solve the problem and the patient may not.[41] Make sure that the connection between the cue and the solution is clear. Ask yourself, "How will the patient use this cue?"
   e. Teach the patient to utilize "chaining" of the activity, i.e., breaking it down into functional components.
   f. Have the patient describe how he would define and carry out a given problem.[193] Have him continue the process by describing how he is doing something as he is doing it.[66] Progress from external environmental cues to internal cues by subvocalization (i.e., the patient tells himself what he's doing as he's doing it).
   g. Have the patient plan the step in problem solution before doing it.
   h. Have the patient label the steps of the task to make them more meaningful, therefore increasing his memory of them.[66]
2. In the belief that improvement in one task will transfer into another, have the patient engage in activites such as anagrams, puzzles, and block designs.
3. Some clinicians advocate the use of videogames and computers for the remediation of problem solving skills.
4. Utilizing a multimodality approach, apply several of the treatment strategies described.

Acalculia

Acalculia, or the inability to perform calculations, is associated with a loss of one or more component skills depending on the location of the lesion. The deficit may be related to poor comprehension of the number structure or specifically to arithmetic operations.[58] Disturbances may be related to alexia or agraphia (impaired ability to read or write), or a disorder of spatial organization, or may be at least partially independent from these two impairments.[111,147,152]

Lesion site: right or left hemisphere — temporal, parietal, or occipital lobes.

Note: A deficit may be seen in isolation or in association with other deficits (Gerstmann's syndrome).[152]

Evaluation of Acalculia

TEST NO. 1: Wechsler Adult Intelligence Scale (WAIS) — Arithmetic Subscale[235]

Description: This is a 14 item timed test consisting of word problems, which range from simple to complex operations.

Scoring: Standardized.

To improve validity, rule out decreased attention, oculomotor skills, and aphasia as causes of poor performance.

TEST NO. 2: Functional Calculations Evaluation

Description: An evaluation can be developed that contains test items for recognition of numbers, simple mathematical operations, and complex mathematical operations, including concepts associated with these operations.[147,152] Test items that are functionally oriented should be incorporated into the evaluation, e.g., coin recognition, calculating change, check writing, or budgeting.

Scoring: Nonstandardized. The clinician measures the patient's level of performance on each category of tasks described.

To improve validity, rule out poor visual attentiveness and oculomotor skills, decreased attention, problem solving, mental inflexibility, and aphasia as causes of poor performance.

Treatment of Acalculia

1. In the belief that improvement in one task will transfer into another, have the patient perform calculation tasks involving number recognition and various levels of addition, subtraction, division, and mulitiplication. Problems should progress from one step operations to multiple step operations as the patient improves.

2. Utilizing a functional approach, incorporate money handling, purchasing, check writing, and budgeting activities into the treatment program.
3. Some clinicians advocate the use of computers for the remediation of acalculia.
4. Utilizing a multimodality approach, apply several of the treatment strategies described.

CHAPTER IX

Factors That Influence the Patient's Cognitive Skills

Many areas of skill have an influence on the patient's cognitive skills. Aphasia, sensory loss, and visual and perceptual deficits can all complicate or interfere with the patient's cognitive abilities. Detailed information about these areas has been presented elsewhere in this book. In addition to these areas, age and environment can influence the patient's cognitive (and perceptual) skills. The effects of age and environment on cognition are described in this section.

Relationship of Age to Perceptual and Cognitive Evaluation and Treatment

The incidence of stroke escalates rapidly with advancing age, from 3.3 per 100,000 persons under 35 to 1800 or more in those 85 years old or older.[199] One study reports that, of 578 patients who had sustained strokes, 76.5 percent were between the ages of 60 and 99 years.[175] A similar study reports that 81 percent of the stroke population were between 65 and 74 years of age and 92.5 percent were between 75 and 84 years.[199]

Despite research and clinical evidence that the majority of the patients who sustain strokes are elderly, functional neurological changes that occur as the result of normal aging are rarely taken into account during perceptual and cognitive evaluation and treatment. The following section is an attempt to acquaint the reader with the major changes related to the normal aging process that may affect perceptual and cognitive functioning. For more detailed information about aging, the reader is referred to references 8, 22, 35, 49, 92, 94, 96, 134, 142, 147, and 188.

Sensory Loss

Vision. Visual acuity and adaptability decline with age.[92,191,226] Decreased depth perception and peripheral vision may also occur.[49] Changes occur in the cornea, pupil, iris, lens, vitreous, and ciliary muscles of the eyes.[49,92,94,191] These changes are summarized in Figure 9-1.

Audition. Hearing losses caused by aging are always bilateral and usually symmetrical.[188] Age related changes might include decreased inner ear function, thickening of the tympanic membrane, loss of elasticity of the ossicular chain, and atrophy of the cochlea or organ of Corti.[49,188] As a result of the structural changes of the auditory system, any or all of the following functional changes might occur:
1. High frequency loss
2. All frequency loss
3. Neural problems that result in decreased speech comprehension and discrimination

Figure 9-1. Changes in the Visual System Associated with Age

Structural Component	Age Related Change	Functional Implications
Cornea	1. Appearance change	Loss of luster, limited amount of fluid bathing the cornea
	2. Accumulation of lipids	Increased astigmatism with increased blurred vision (independent of near- or farsightedness)
Iris	Decreased permeability	May contribute to glaucoma
Ciliary muscle	Atrophy of muscle	Decreased mobility of the lens which causes decreased muscle effectiveness
Pupil	1. Decreased pupil size	Restricted amount of light reaching retina; difficulty in seeing dark objects or objects in dim light
	2. Decreased pupillary reflex	Decreased dark adaptation and recovery from glare
Lens	1. Lens growth	Decreased accommodative ability
	2. Decreased refractive index of lenses	Uneven refracture properties, which can result in double vision in one eye
	3. Yellowing	Reduces amount of light reaching retina and changes light composition; alters color vision
Vitreous	Contracts	May separate from retina (the retina itself may also detach)

4. Problems in determining the source of a sound
5. Distortion of environmental sound
6. Difficulty hearing in the presence of background noise
7. Impaired intellectual functioning

Remaining Sensory Systems. Research has indicated that in at least a portion of the elderly population, there is a reduced sensitivity to taste, smell, touch, vibration, temperature, kinesthesia, and pain.[92]

Autonomic Nervous System

Age related changes in the hypothalamus have been observed and seem to result in decreased maintenance of homeostasis.[82,96]

Age related changes occur in the metabolism and regulatory mechanisms of an organism. Aging is "characterized by a progressive decrease in the intensity of adaptive processes."[90] It is believed that with aging, autonomic nervous system changes take place throughout all aspects of the system. These changes lead to shifts in the reflectory regulation of inner organs, to a decrease in the organism's adaptive capacities, to a decrease in the reliability of homeostatic regulatory mechanisms, to an easier disruption of regulatory mechanisms, and to the development of disorders in old age.[96]

Perception

In view of the close relationship between vision and perception, it can be expected that age related visual changes will influence perceptual abilities in the elderly. For example, the decreased accommodative power and poor lens transmissiveness previously described can in turn affect distance vision, sensitivity to glare, and depth and color perception.[94] Losses in acuity and susceptibility to glare could also affect the ability to use monocular cues for distance perception.[94] Visual closure, or part-whole perception, may also be deficient.[94] The quality of stereopsis depends on brightness and contrast. Therefore, any age related process that reduces retinal illumination would impair binocular depth perception.[94]

In addition to distance, depth, and color perception, the elderly's visual fields may be altered. This age related change involves the retina and the nervous system in general. Age related circulatory changes can cause a metabolic change in the retina, which in turn is reflected by changes in the size of the visual field.[94]

Cognition

Research has indicated that decreased brain weight and volume and a decrease in the cells of the cerebral cortex occur with age.[38,45] Since the cerebral cortex is intricately involved with higher intellectual functioning, cognitive and behavioral changes might be expected with age. The following is an overview of documented age related cognitive impairments.

The documentation of decreased memory of one type or another in the elderly is abundant.[8,22,35,134,142,192,197,198] Some authors believe that age related memory loss is primarily a storage and retrieval problem. Others believe that nonverbal memory is a particular problem for the elderly, and that they will benefit from the use of verbal cues to improve their performance.[142,198] Still others believe age related memory impairment to be due to the inefficient use of learning strategies.[8,147] For example, the elderly do not use repetition, visual imagery, verbal mediation, association encoding, mnemonics, or organization strategies as often or as effectively as younger individuals.[8,22,147] Inefficient use of all or any of these strategies means that the retrieval cues are minimal.[8] Retrieval deficits in the elderly in association with new information do not appear to generalize to very old memory.

A generalized slowing of cognitive processes and reaction time in the elderly has also been documented.[33,177] There is diminished ability for abstract and complex conceptualization, and poor mental flexibility.[92,147] These deficits, along with decreased memory, can cause difficulty in adapting to new situations, solving novel problems, and changing from one mental set to another.[92,147] There is indeed documentation of poor problem solving ability among the elderly.[5,92,133,193,245]

Implications for Evaluation

Some of the age related deficits described in this section may or may not be present in a given individual. It is vital for the occupational therapist to obtain a clear picture of the stroke patient's premorbid status prior to perceptual or cognitive evaluation and treatment. Vision should be evaluated prior to testing, and measures that involve small visual stimuli should be avoided if possible. Responses that require fine color discrimination, especially in the blue spectrum, may be invalid.[42] One should use color contrasts, an increased amount of light, and clean prescription glasses when indicated. Determine the patient's hearing acuity. Evaluate the effects of modifying your voice, identify the best position to sit or stand to reinforce what is said, and make sure that the patient's hearing aid is clean.[49] Consult vision and hearing experts when there is a question.

Always remember that for the elderly testing is often a threatening experience. The fear of testing may in fact limit their risk taking and inhibit their response. Consider the environment when testing: the elderly are more easily distracted by irrelevant stimuli than younger individuals.[70]

Finally, consider fatigue in testing.[8,147] Mental fatigue at any age can cause various sensory and perceptual changes, slowed and disorganized performance, and perhaps short term memory impairment.[70]

Implications in Treatment

The areas to consider for evaluation are also applicable to treatment. In addition, the therapist should limit redundant and extraneous information and treat in a nondistracting environment.[8,198] Repetition and practice are indicated because the elderly (along with the young) can benefit from this.[8] Allow sufficient time for the patient to respond and utilize cues that will most benefit the patient, e.g., verbal, visual, touch, or movement.

In addition to practice and cuing, the elderly patient who has sustained a stroke can benefit from controlled sensory stimulation and sensory integrative techniques.[179] These treatment approaches are covered in detail in Chapter I.

Environmental Influence on Cognition

As described in the section on the sensory integrative approach to treatment, an individual's interaction with his surroundings is crucial to normal development and the maintenance of health. The central nervous system is an open feedback system, which continually reacts to external influences and events.[65] The brain, even in a pathological state, as in the case of cerebral vascular disease, continues to react to environmental influences. Theoretically, if an individual can perceive stimulation from the environment, he may be able subsequently to change his behavior in response to these environmental changes.

It is crucial to incorporate the concept of environmental influence on behavior into the cognitive remediation program for the stroke patient. Cognitive rehabilitation must be concerned with problems and alterations of environment to facilitate improved function. By therapeutically altering the environment, the patient can be helped to learn mental strategies for task performance and gradually progress to more difficult tasks.[37]

Therapeutic environmental alteration can range from specific physical changes to changes in the structuring of tasks and in the amount of feedback the therapist gives the patient during an activity. An example of actual physical changes in an environment would be the treatment of a distractable patient in an uncluttered quiet room with few physical distractions. The use of structuring of tasks can also be applied to the distractable patient. Providing a great deal of structure for the patient during the activity will decrease his distractable behavior. As the patient masters an activity, he can progress to a more normal environment with less structure provided.[159]

The technique of feedback or environmental "cuing" is key to improved cognitive function. Cuing includes any alteration of the instructions or conditions of a task made to improve patient functioning.[92] Environmental cuing can range from feedback, utilizing any sensory system, to the use of tokens or progress charts placed over the patient's bed. Altering the amount, duration, and complexity and type of cuing utilized can have a direct effect on the patient's performance.[159] If a patient is not performing well on a particular task, the reason may lie in the type or amount of cuing that was provided by the therapist. The therapist should always be cognizant of the effect of cuing on the patient's performance, changing the cuing as often as necessary for optimal performance.

The ultimate goal of cognitive rehabilitation is the internalization of cuing strategies or, at a minimum, the reduced need for external environmental cuing for successful functioning. The patient with a memory problem, for instance, should learn to cue himself to remember important information necessary for daily functioning, and the inattentive patient should progress to being able to cue himself to pay attention. Figure 9-2 summarizes the

**Figure 9-2. Use of Environment in Cognitive Rehabilitation
Patient Progression**

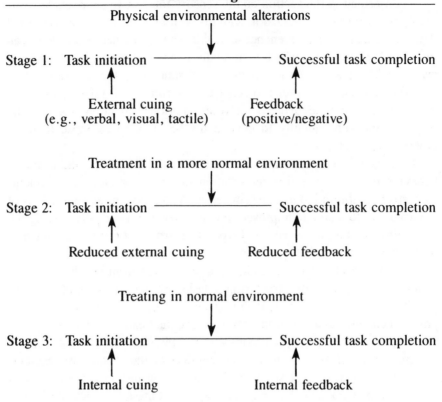

Physical environmental alterations

Stage 1: Task initiation ——————— Successful task completion

External cuing   Feedback
(e.g., verbal, visual, tactile)   (positive/negative)

Treatment in a more normal environment

Stage 2: Task initiation ——————— Successful task completion

Reduced external cuing   Reduced feedback

Treating in normal environment

Stage 3: Task initiation ——————— Successful task completion

Internal cuing   Internal feedback

desired patient progression in cognitive rehabilitation as it relates to use of environment as a therapeutic tool.

CHAPTER X

The Use of Computers in Cognitive Retraining

The application of computer technology to health care has increased rapidly in recent years. Probably the most recent use of computers in health care has been in direct patient treatment. In a recent survey of 16 facilities conducted by St. Joseph Hospital in New Mexico, 15 respondents acknowledged the use of computers in patient care.[218] Such use can range from prevocational applications, to environmental control, to visual, perceptual, or cognitive retraining.[172,232] The specific use of the computer in the retraining of cognitive skills will be described in this section.

A review of the literature and correspondence with experts in the field reveal a mixture of attitudes toward the use of computers in patient care. Smith states that personal computers give handicapped patients access to much more of the world than has been possible before.[42,214] Bracy supports this idea of environmental interaction in stating that in order to function independently, the injured patient must regain the ability to interact with the environment.[42] He must deal with new situations, plan and make decisions, and act on these decisions. Bracy states that computers are good tools for developing the fundamental skills needed for such activity.

Gianutsos applauds the use of computers for cognitive retraining as a means of increasing our capacity for precision, flexibility, and efficiency.[102] She goes on to state that computer retraining can be used to carry out many of the tedious tasks associated with cognitive retraining. Recent technological advances have made possible the sale of less expensive computers, making them a potentially highly cost-effective rehabilitation tool.[212] Additional advantages of computers include the immediate and consistent feedback, short presentation times, standardization of training, objectivity, and convenient data storage.[154,181,182]

Several authors are more cautious with their accolades for computer based cognitive retraining. Parente states that this retraining may improve eye-hand coordination, attention, and concentration but not the ability to retrieve information from memory.[181] The use of videogames is described as an appropriate adjunct to cognitive remediation, but not as a replacement for human intervention and contact.[155]

Wilson supports this notion in stating that it is important to remember that the computer is just a tool, which can be used in assisting the learning process.[241]

Several disadvantages have been identified with the use of computers in cognitive retraining. Early videogames, for instance, tended to be based on aggressive themes of attacking, killing, or blowing up, which were offensive to some patients.[154] Limitations in software design and availability, decreased ease of patient use, and computer anxiety were also identified as disadvantages of this approach.[182] In addition, the computer may be unnecessary for simple cognitive retraining.[181]

The early stage of development of computer based cognitive retraining is manifest by the paucity of documented controlled studies describing its effect. Lynch reflects the state of the art well when he notes that despite the enormous number of videogame machines and personal computers in use today, there are surprisingly few published research studies dealing with the effects of videogame training upon cognitive, perceptual motor, or practical activities of daily living such as driving and dressing.[154]

Indeed, an extensive literature search and correspondence with experts in the field yielded little information, for the primary emphasis has been placed on case presentations or program descriptions.[42,153,254] These few documented studies are presented in the following paragraphs.

Sivak, Hill, and Olson provided four brain damaged patients (two suffering strokes and two with head injuries) with 10 hours (six sessions over two weeks) of computer based cognitive retraining.[212] The WAIS picture completion, picture arrangement, and block design subtests, a cancellation task, the Rey-Osterrieth complex figure test, and the trailmaking and symbol digit modalities tests were all given before and after training. The subjects were trained with an Apple II+ on programs that included simple visual reaction, visual reaction-stimulus discrimination, mazes, cube-in-a-box, paddleball, search, simple search, and the like. Following training, two subjects showed improvement in several perceptual tests, and the remaining two showed improvement in a limited number of tests. These authors interpreted their study as showing positive results requiring further study.

Parente conducted computer based cognitive retraining with adult patients with head injuries to improve memory.[181] His patients utilized an inexpensive microcomputer (Texas Instruments TI99/4A) for daily in-home practice for approximately two to four hours per day. He utilized programs that teach organizational and encoding skills as a basis for improved memory. This computer retraining was associated with an increase in standardized memory scores. Discussions with patients and family members indicated improved memory in daily life. Parente noted that major improvement may take six to 12 months and that significant improvement usually occurs within 10 sessions. Parente has found computer based retraining to be particularly useful for improving efficiency and teaching skills that will generalize.[181]

Lynch describes positive effects of computer based training in his work with patients sustaining cerebrovascular accidents, tumors, Alzheimer's disease, and brain trauma.[153] These effects include stimulation (as a means of sustaining attention and motivation) and memory enhancement (words, visual spatial, patterns, sequences), and its use as a substitute for other games (cards, chess). Lynch notes that additional benefits of computer use are that the programs can provide additional cues and clarification and can continually adjust to the patient's performance.

Bracy utilizes computer based training with brain damaged patients to enhance sensory input, increase the patient's ability to selectively attend and maintain that attention for extended periods, and aid in making decisions.[42] Bracy's program is an outpatient home based program. He sees his patients once a week, and the remaining computer time is spent by the patient at home. The patient practices approximately three times a day for a total of one to five hours per day. Retraining lasts six to 12 months.

Gracey utilizes computer assisted training with head injured patients to increase attentional skills, problem solving, visual memory, auditory discrimination, and visual scanning.[110] An Apple II microcomputer is utilized, and patients are encouraged to use it during nonstructured time. Gracey states that patients appear to be responsive to the program and has noted gains in selective attention, improved response time, and increased self-esteem.

Several problems are evident in regard to the studies described. One of the most obvious limitations is small sample size. In addition, although there has been occasional use of standardized measures, the majority of the conclusions have been based on clinical observations or conversations with the patient or his family. There is no doubt that these qualitative measures are important, especially in clinical practice; however, quantitative measures are required in clinical research. Other limitations of the described studies are the timing and duration of cognitive retraining. All studies have dealt with outpatients during a nonacute stage of recovery. In most instances training involves long hours, mostly by the patient at home. We were unable to find even one program description that dealt with inpatients during the acute stage of recovery.

Probably one of the greatest problems with available documented studies is the lack of use of control groups. When there is no comparison group that is not receiving the benefit of a particular treatment, it is difficult to adequately test the efficacy of this treatment.

Despite the shortcomings of the present research documentation of computer use in cognitive retraining, the clinical experience of experts in the field indicates a strong potential for successful application. In order to maximize this potential, it is important that the therapist choose computer software appropriately. Lynch[153] assists the therapist by providing some basic guidelines related to the mechanics of the computer equipment:

1. Games should be simple and uncluttered.

2. Games should contain low basic performance levels as well as high ceilings.

3. Games should not include much, if any, keyboard input. A joystick, light pen, or space bar should be available for the patient to respond.

4. Use programs that continually adjust to the patient's performance.

5. Use large print letters and numbers.

6. Be aware of the patient's emotional response.

7. Select tools that are simple to use, e.g., cartridges or modules rather than cassettes.

Wilson[241] has provided specific guidelines for software selection that analyze the specific components or format of a given program. She suggests asking the following questions:

1. Is the level of difficulty or complexity of the items controlled and consistent?

2. Can you enter your own items into the program in addition to using only the preprogramed items?

3. Are instructions concise and easy to follow?

4. Is the response format consistent so that the learner does not become confused?

5. Is the content accurate? Are there any parts of the program that are demeaning?

6. How much supervision, if any, is needed for the patient to run the program?

7. What type of feedback is supplied to the user?

8. What variables can you control (e.g., the length of time the stimulus is displayed, the time that elapses until the patient must respond, the level of difficulty, the speed of task performance, the size of the letters, and the time and type of reinforcement)?

9. How are error responses represented?

10. How are data kept and reported to you?

11. Does the program provide instructions on the screen?[241]

In addition to general guidelines, it is important for the therapist to remain abreast of state of the art software. Wilson has assisted us in this process by developing an annotated bibliography relating to cognitive retraining software (refer to Appendix B).

REFERENCES

1. Acker W: In support of the microcomputer based automated testing: a description of the Maudsley automated psychological screening tests (MAPS). Br J Alcohol Alcoholism, 15:144-147, 1980.

2. Adams GF: Treatment of hemiplegia complicated by sensory defects. Physiotherapy 52:345-349, 1966.

3. Anderson E, Choy E: Parietal lobe syndromes in hemiplegia, a program for treatment. Am J Occup Ther 24:13-18, 1970.

4. Archibald YM, Wepman JM: Language disturbance and non-verbal cognitive performance in eight patients following injury to the right hemisphere. Brain 91:117-129, 1968.

5. Arenberg D: A longitudinal study of problem solving in adults. J Gerontol 29:656-658, 1974.

6. Arenberg D: Concept problem solving in young and old adults. J Gerontol 23:279-282, 1968.

7. Arenberg D: The effects of auditory augmentation on visual retention for young and old adults. J Gerontol 32:192-195, 1977.

8. Arenberg D, Robertson-Tchabo E: Learning and aging. In Birren J, Schaie K (eds.): Handbook of the Psychology of Aging. New York, Von Reinhold Co., 1977, pp. 421-449.

9. Atkinson RC, Shiffrin RM: The control of short-term memory. Sci Am 225(2):82-89, 1971.

10. Ayres AJ: Institute on Sensory Integrative Dysfunction and Learning Disabilities. Lecture, Sheraton-Boston, October 13-14, 1972.

11. Ayres AJ: Perception of space of adult hemiplegic patients. Arch Phys Med 43:552-555, 1962.

12. Ayres AJ: Sensory Integration and Learning Disorders. Los Angeles, Western Psychological Services, 1980.

13. Ayres AJ: Sensory Integration and the Child. Los Angeles, Western Psychological Services, 1980.

14. Ayres AJ: Southern California Sensory Integration Tests. Los Angeles, Western Psychological Services, 1972.

15. Bach-y-Rita P: Recovery of Function: Theoretical Considerations for Brain Injury Rehabilitation. Bern, Hans Huber Publishers, 1980.

16. Baddeley AD: Memory theory and memory therapy. In Wilson BA, Moffat N (eds.): Clinical Management of Memory Problems. Rockville, Maryland, Aspen Publishers, 1984, pp. 5-27.

17. Baillet R, Blood K, Bach-y-Rita P: Visual field rehabilitation in the cortically blind. J Neurol Neurosurg Psychiat (to be published).

18. Baker-Nobles L, Bink MP: Sensory integration in the rehabilitation of blind adults. Am J Occup Ther 33(9):559-564, 1979.

19. Balts P, Schaie K: On the plasticity of intelligence in adulthood and old age. Am Psychol 720-725, October 1976.

20. Baltes P, Warner Schaie K: The myth of the twilight years: aging and IQ. Psychol Today 35-40, March 1974.

21. Bannister R: Brain's Clinical Neurology. London, Oxford University Press, 1973.

22. Bartus RT: Effects of aging on visual memory, sensory processing and discrimination learning in a nonhuman primate. In Ordy JM, Bizzle KR (eds.): Aging. Vol. 10. Sensory Systems and Communications in the Elderly. New York, Raven Press, 1979.

23. Baum B: The establishment of reliability and validity of a perceptual evaluation on a sample of adult head trauma patients. Thesis, University of Southern California, December 1981.

24. Baum B, Hall K: Relationship between constructional praxis and dressing in the head injured adult. Am J Occup Ther 35(7):438-442, 1981.

25. Bender M: Comments on the physiology and pathology of eye movements in the vertical plane. J Nerv Ment Dis 130:456-466, 1960.

26. Bennett-Levy J, Powell G: The subjective memory questionnaire (SMQ). An investigation into the self-reporting of "real-life" memory skills. Br J Soc Clin Psychol 19:177-188, 1980.

27. Benton A: Right-Left Discrimination and Finger Localization. New York, Harper Bros., 1959.

28. Benton AL, Fogel ML: Three-dimensional constructional praxis, a clinical test. Arch Neurol 7:347-354, 1962.

29. Ben-Yishay Y, Diller L: Rehabilitation of cognitive and perceptual defects in people with traumatic brain damage. Int J Rehab Res 4(2):208-210, 1981.

30. Ben-Yishay Y, et al.: Working Approaches to Remediation of Cognitive Deficits in Brain Damaged Persons. Rehabilitaton Monograph 64. New York, New York University Medical Center, April 1982.

31. Ben-Yishay Y, et al.: Working Approaches to Remediation of Cognitive Deficits in Brain Damaged Persons. Rehabilitation Monograph 62. New York, New York University Medical Center, May 1981.

32. Bergmann K: A visual tracking machine. Am J Occup Ther 31(7):421-424, 1977.

33. Birnbaum MH: Esotropia, exotropia and cognitive/perceptual style. J Am Optom Assoc 52(8):635-639, 1981.

34. Birren J, Morrison D: Analysis of the WAIS subtests in relation to age and education. J Gerontol 16:363-369, 1961.

35. Birren J, Renner V: Research on the psychology of aging: principles and experimentation. In Birren J, Schaie K (eds.): Handbook of the Psychology of Aging. New York, Von Nostrand Reinhold Co., 1977.

36. Bobath B: Adult Hemiplegia, Evaluation and Treatment. London, William Hennemann Medical Books Ltd., 1978.

37. Bolger J: Cognitive retraining: a developmental approach. Clin Neuropsychol 4:66-70, 1982.

38. Bondareff W: The neural basis of aging. In Birren J, Schaie K (eds.): Handbook of the Psychology of Aging. New York, Von Nostrand Reinhold Co., 1977.

39. Boone D, Landes B: Left-right discrimination in hemiplegic patients. Arch Phys Med 49:533-537, 1968.

40. Batwinick J, Storandt M: Recall and recognition of old information in relation to age and sex. J Gerontol 35(1):70-76, 1980.

41. Bourne LE, Dominowski RL, Loftus EF: Cognitive Processes. Englewood Cliffs, New Jersey, Prentice-Hall, Inc.,1979.

42. Bracy O: Computer based cognitive rehabilitation. Cognit Rehab 1(1):7-8, 1983.

43. Breines E. Perception: Its Development and Recapitulation. Princeton, Geri-Rehab, 1981.

44. Brodal A: Neurological Anatomy (3rd edition). New York, Oxford University Press, 1981.

45. Brody H, Vijayashankar N: Anatomical changes in the nervous system. In Finch CE, Hayfbeck L (eds.): Handbook of the Biology of Aging. New York, Van Nostrand Reinhold Co., 1977.

46. Brooks N, Lincoln NB: Assessment for rehabilitation. In Wilson BA, Moffat N (eds.): Clinical Management of Memory Problems. Rockville, Maryland, Aspen Publishers, 1984.

47. Brown J: Aphasia, Apraxia and Agnosia, Clinical and Theoretical Aspects. Springfield, Illinois, Charles C Thomas Publ., 1972.

48. Burt M: Perceptual deficits in hemiplegia. Am J Nurs 70:1026-1029, 1970.

49. Buseck S, Shields E: Aging: sensory losses. Available from American Journal of Nursing Co., Educational Services Division, 555 W. 57th Street, New York, New York. (Study guide and videotape.)

50. Butters N, Barton M: Effect of parietal lobe damage on the performance of reversible operations in space. Neuropsychologia 8:205-214, 1970.

51. Butters N, Barton M, Brody BA: Role of the right parietal lobe in the mediation of cross-modal associations and reversible operations in space. Cortex 6:174-190, 1970.

52. Butters N, Brody BA: The role of the left parietal lobe in the mediation of intra- and cross-modal associations. Cortex 4:328-343, 1968.

53. Butters N, Samuels I, Goodglass H, Brody B: Short-term visual and auditory memory disorders after parietal and frontal lobe damage. Unpublished data.

54. Caramazam, et al.: Right hemisphere damage and verbal problem solving behavior. Brain Language 3:41-46, 1976.

55. Carter L, Cartioz J, Languirand M, Bernard MA: Cognitive skill remediation in stroke and non-stroke elderly. Clin Neuropsychol 2(3):109-113, 1980.

56. Carter L, Howard B, O'Neil W.: Effectiveness of cognitive skill remediation in acute stroke patients. Am J Occup Ther 37(5):320-326, 1983.

57. Cermak L: Imagery as an aid to retrieval for Korsakoff patients. Cortex 11:163-169, 1975.

58. Christenson AL: Luria's Neuropsychological Investigation. New York, Spectrum Publications, 1975.

59. Chusid JG: Correlative Neuroanatomy and Functional Neurology (17th edition). Los Altos, California, Lange Medical Publications, 1979.

60. Chusid JG, McDonald JJ: Correlative Neuroanatomy and Functional Neurology (19th edition). Los Altos, California, Lange Medical Publications, 1985.

61. Clawson-Sanders J, Sterns H, Smith M, Sanders R: Modification of concept identification performance in older adults. Devel Psychol 11(6): 824-829, 1975.

62. Cohen SA: A dynamic theory of vision. J Devel Reading, 6(1):15-25, 1962.

63. Coltheart M, Lea CD, Thompson K: In defense of iconic memory. Quart J Exp Psychol 26:633-641, 1974.

64. Craik F: Human memory. Ann Rev Psychol 30: 63-102, 1979.

65. Craine JF: Principles of cognitive rehabilitation. In Trexler LE (ed.): Cognitive Rehabilitation: Conceptualization and Intervention. New York, Plenum Press, 1982.

66. Craine J: The retraining of frontal lobe dysfunction. In Trexler LE (ed.): Cognitive Rehabilitation: Conceptualization and Intervention. New York, Plenum Press, 1982.

67. Craine JF, Gudeman HE: The Rehabilitation of Brain Functions: Principles, Procedures and Techniques of Neurotraining. Springfield, Illinois, Charles C Thomas Publ., 1981.

68. Cratty BJ: Movement Behavior and Motor Learning (2nd edition). Philadelphia, Lea & Febiger, 1967.

69. Critchley M: The Parietal Lobes. London, Edward Arnold Co., 1953.

70. Crook T: Psychometric assessment in the elderly. In Raskin A, Javick L (eds.): Psychiatric Symptoms and Cognitive Loss in the Elderly. New York, Hemisphere Publishing Co., 1979, pp. 207-220.

71. Crosson B, Bruenning W: An individualized memory retraining program after closed-head injury: a single-case study. J Clin Neuropsychol 6(3):287-301, 1984.

72. Crovitz H: Memory retraining in brain damaged patients: the airplane list. Cortex 15:131-134, 1979.

73. Crovitz HF, Harvey MT, Horn RW: Problems in the acquisition of imagery mnemonics: three brain damaged cases. Cortex, 225-234, 1979.

74. Dahlen A, Fex S, Henriksson NG, Pyikko I: Dyspraxia of speech and eye motility. Acta Otolaryngol 89:144-151, 1980.

75. Darley FL: Diagnosis and Appraisal of Communication Disorders. Englewood Cliffs, New Jersey, Prentice-Hall, Inc., 1964.

76. Davies PM: Steps to Follow—A Guide to the Treatment of Adult Hemiplegia. Berlin, Springer-Verlag, 1985.

77. Delisa J, Meller R, Melnick R, Mikulic M: Stroke rehabilitation. Part 1. Cognitive deficits and prediction of outcome. AFP 207-214, November 1982.

78. Denny-Brown D: The nature of apraxia. J Nerv Ment Dis 126:9-32, 1958.

79. DeRenzi E, Faglioni P: The relationship between visuo-spatial impairment and construction. Cortex 3:327-342, 1967.

80. DeRenzi E, Faglioni P, Previdi P. Spatial memory and hemispheric locus of lesion. Cortex 13:424-433, 1978.

81. DeRenzi E, Spinnler H: The influence of verbal and non-verbal defects on visual memory tasks. Cortex 2:322-335, 1966.

82. Diamond MC: The aging brain: some enlightening and optimistic results. Am Scient 66:66-71, 1978.

83. Diller L: A model for cognitive retraining in rehabilitation. Clin Psychol 29(2):13-15, 1978.

84. Diller L: Studies in Cognition and Rehabilitation in Hemiplegia. Research grant RD-2666-P. New York, Institute of Rehabilitation Medicine, July 1971.

85. Diller L, Gordon W: Interventions for cognitive deficits in brain-injured adults. J Consult Clin Psychol 49(6):822-834, 1981.

86. Diller L, Weinberg J: Differential aspects of attention in brain damaged persons. Percept Motor Skills 35:71-81, 1972.

87. Ditchburn R: Eye Movements and Visual Perception. Oxford, Claredon Press, 1973.

88. Dodd DH, White RM: Cognition: Mental Structures and Processes. Boston, Allyn & Bacon, Inc., 1980.

89. Doehring DG, Reitan RM, Klove H: Changes in patterns of intelligence test performance associated with homonymous visual field defects. J Nerv Ment Dis 132:227-233, 1961.

90. Drachman D, Leavitt J: Memory impairment in the aged: storage vs. retrieval deficit. J Exp Psychol 93(2):302-308, 1972.

91. Fiebert IM, Brown E: Vestibular stimulation to improve ambulation after a cerebral vascular accident. Phys Ther 59(4):423-426, 1979.

92. Filskov S, Boll T: Handbook of Clinical Neuropsychology. New York, John Wiley & Sons, Inc., 1981.

93. Fox JVD: Effect of cutaneous stimulation on performance of hemiplegic adults on selected tests of perception. Thesis, University of Southern California, 1963.

94. Fozard J, Wolf E, Bell B, McFarland R, Podolsky S: Visual perception and communication. In Birren J, Schaie K (eds.): Handbook of Psychology of Aging. New York, Van Nostrand Reinhold Co, 1977.

95. Frankenberg WK, Dodds JB: Denver Developmental Screening Test. Denver, Ladoca Project and Publishing Foundation, Inc., 1970 (revised).

96. Frolkis V: Aging of the autonomic nervous system. In Birren J, Schaie K (eds.): Handbook of the Psychology of Aging. New York, Von Nostrand Reinhold Co., 1977.

97. Frostig M: Developmental Test of Visual Perception. Palo Alto, Consulting Psychologists Press, 1966 (revised).

98. Frostig M, Horne D: Frostig Program for the Development of Visual Perception (revised edition). Chicago, Follett Publishing Co., 1973.

99. Frostig M, Maslow P, Lefever DW, Whittlesey JRB: The Marianne Frostig Developmental Test of Visual Perception, 1963 Standardization. Palo Alto, Consulting Psychologists Press, 1964.

100. Gardner E: Fundamentals of Neurology. Philadelphia, W.B. Saunders Company, 1968.

101. Gainotti G, Tiacci C: Patterns of drawing disability in right and left hemispheric patients. Neuropsychologia 8:379-384, 1970.

102. Gianutsos R: What is cognitive rehabilitation? J Rehab 36-40, July/Aug/Sept 1980.

103. Geschwind N: Late changes in the central nervous system; an overview. In Stein D, Rosen J, Bulters N (eds.): Plasticity and Recovery of Function in the Central Nervous System. New York, Academic Press, Inc., 1974.

104. Glasgow RE, Zeiss RA, Barrera JR, Lewinsohn PM: Case studies on remediating memory deficits in brain-damaged individuals. J Clin Psychol 33(4):1049-1054, 1977.

105. Gloning K, Hoff H: Cerebral localization of disorders of higher nervous activity. In Vinken PH, Bruyn GW (eds.): Handbook of Clinical Neurology. Vol. 3. Disorders of Higher Nervous Activity. New York, John Wiley & Sons, Inc., 1969.

106. Golden C, Ariel R, McKay S, Wilkening G, Wolf B, MacInnes W: The Luria-Nebraska neuropsychological battery: theoretical orientation and comment. J Consult Clin Psychol 50(2):291-300, 1982.

107. Goldman H: Improvement in double simultaneous stimulation perception in hemiplegic patients. Arch Phys Med 47:681-687, 1966.

108. Goodenough F, Harris D: Goodenough-Harris Drawing Test. New York, Harcourt, Brace & World, 1963.

109. Goodglass H, Kaplan E: The Assessment of Aphasia and Related Disorders. Philadelphia, Lea & Febiger, 1972.

110. Gracy S: Computer assisted therapy for brain injured patients—a team approach. Phys Disab Spec Inter Sect Newsletter 7(2):4, 1984.

111. Grafman J, Passafuime D, Faglioni P, Boller F: Calculation disturbances in adults with focal hemispheric damage. Cortex 18:37-50, 1982.

112. Gregory ME, Aitkin JA: Assessment of parietal lobe function in hemiplegia. Occup Ther 34:9-17, 1971.

113. Gronwell D, Wrightson P: Memory and information processing capacity after closed head injury. J Neurol Neurosurg Psychiat 44:889-895, 1981.

114. Hague HR: An investigation of abstract behavior in patients with cerebral vascular accidents. Am J Occup Ther 13:83-87, 1959.

115. Halperin E, Cohen BS: Perceptual-motor dysfunction, stumbling block to rehabilitation. Maryland Med J 20:139-141, 1971.

116. Harrington DO: The Visual Fields (4th edition). St. Louis, The C.V. Mosby Co., 1976.

117. Harris J: Memory aids people use: two interview studies. Mem Cognit 8(1):31-36, 1980.

118. Harris J: Methods of improving memory. In Wilson BA, Moffat N (eds.): Clinical Management of Memory Problems. Rockville, Maryland, Aspen Publishers, 1984.

119. Harris JE, Sunderland A: A brief survey of the management of memory disorders in rehabilitation units in Britain. Int Rehab Med 3:206-109, 1981.

120. Heaton JM: The Eye. Philadelphia, J.B. Lippincott Company, 1968.

121. Hecaen H, Assal G: A comparison of constructive deficits following right and left hemispheric lesions. Neuropsychologia 8:289-303, 1970.

122. Hecaen H, Penfield W, Bertrand C, Malmo R: The syndrome of apractognosis due to lesions of the minor cerebral hemisphere. Arch Neurol Psychiat 75:400-434, 1956.

123. Heilman K, Velestrein E: Frontal lobe neglect in man. Neurology 22:660-664, 1972.

124. Hemmingson R, Mejcholm B, Boysen G, Engell HC: Intellectual function in patients with transient ischaemic attacks (TIA) or minor stroke. Acta Neurol Scand 66:145-159, 1982.

125. Henderson A, Cermak S: Problems of perceptual deficits in occupational therapy. Class Notes and Handouts, OT 712, Boston University, 1972-1973.

126. Hendrickson H: The vision development process; visual and perceptual aspects for the achieving and underachieving child. Optometric Extension Program Foundation, Special Child, Seattle, Washington, 1969.

127. Holland A: Language Disorders in Adults. Recent Advances. San Diego, College Hill Press, 1984, pp. 177-209.

128. Hopkins HL: Occupational therapy management of cerebrovascular accident and hemiplegia. In Willard H, Spackman C (eds.): Occupational Therapy (4th edition). Philadelphia, J.B. Lippincott Company, 1971.

129. Hoyer W, Rebok G, Svold S: Effects of varying irrelevant information on adult age differences in problem solving. J Gerontol 34(4): 553-560, 1979.

130. Hultsch D: Adult age differences in retrieval: trace dependent and cue-dependent forgetting. Devel Psychol 11(2):197-201, 1975.

131. Instructo-Clinic —A Psychophysical Testing Apparatus. Bumpa-Tel, Inc., P.O. Box 611, Cape Gir., Missouri 63701.

132. Isaacs B, Kennie A. The set test as an aid to the detection of dementia in old people. Br J Psychiat 123:467-470, 1973.

133. Jerome EA: Decay of heuristic processes in the aged. In Tibbitts C, Donahue W (eds.): Social and Psychological Aspects of Aging. New York, Columbia University Press, 1962.

134. Kahn RL, Zarit SH, Hilbert NM, Niederehe G: Memory complaints and impairment in the aged. Arch Gen Psychiat 32:1569-1573, 1975.

135. Kenshalo DR: Changes in the vestibular and sonmesthetic systems as a function of age. In Ordy JM, Bizzee KR (eds.): Aging. Vol. 10. Sensory Systems and Communication in the Elderly. New York, Raven Press, 1979.

136. Kephart N: Slow Learner in the Classroom. Columbus, Ohio, Charles E. Merrill Publ. Co, 1960.

137. Kortesz A: Subcortical lesions and verbal apraxia. In Rosenbeck J, McNeil M, Aronson A (eds.): Apraxia of Speech. San Diego, College Hill Press, 1984.

138. Kinsbourne M: Cognitive deficit and the unity of brain organization: Goldstein's perspective updated. J Commun Dis 24:181-194, 1981.

139. Kirkpatrick S: Development of body scheme. Unpublished data, 1971.

140. Klonoff H, Kennedy M: A comparative study of cognitive functioning in old age. J Gerontol 21:239-243, 1966.

141. Klonoff H, Kennedy M: Memory and perceptual functioning in octogenarians and nonagenarians in the community. J Gerontol 20:328-333, 1965.

142. Kramer N, Farbik L: Assessment of intellectual changes in the elderly. In Raskin A, Jarbik L (eds.): Psychiatric Symptoms and Cognitive Loss in the Elderly. New York, Hemisphere Publ. Co., 1979.

143. Labowie-Vief, Gonda J: Cognitive strategy training and intellectual performance in the elderly. J Gerontol 31(3):327-332, 1967.

144. Layton B: Perceptual noise and aging. Psychol Bull 82:875-883, 1975.

145. Lewinsohn PM, Danaher BG, Kikel S: Visual imagery as a mnemonic aid for brain-injured persons. J Consult Clin Psychol 45(5):717-723, 1977.

146. Lewinsohn PM, Zieler RE, Lilet J, Eyeberg S, Nielson G: Short-term memory. J Compar Physiol Psychol 1072(81):248-255, 1972.

147. Lezak M: Neuropsychological Assessment. New York, Oxford University Press, 1983.

148. Lezak MD: Subtle sequelae of brain damage: perplexity, distractibility and fatigue. Am J Phys Med 57:9-15, 1978.

149. Lieberman S, Cohen AH, Rubin J: NYSOA K-D test. J Am Optom Assoc 54(7):631-637, 1983.

150. Lorenze EJ, Cancro R: Dysfunction in visual perception with hemiplegia, its relation to activities of daily living. Arch Phys Med 43:514-517, 1962.

151. Luria AR: Functional organization of the brain. Sci Am 222:66-72, 1970.

152. Luria AR: Higher Cortical Functions in Man (2nd edition). New York, Basic Books, Inc., 1980.

153. Lynch WJ: The contribution of video games to computer-assisted cognitive training. Presentation at Symposium on Innovative Rehabilitatioin Approaches for the Geriatric Patient, 91st Annual Convention, American Psychological Association, Anaheim, California, August 26-30, 1983.

154. Lynch WJ: The use of electronic games in cognitive rehabilitation. In Trexler LE (ed.): Cognitive Rehabilitation—Conceptualization and Intervention. New York, Plenum Press, 1982.

155. Lynch WT: Video games in the remediation of cognitive and perceptual-motor disorders: experience, problems and prospects. Presented at Symposium on Video Games and Human Development: A Research Agenda for the 80's, Harvard Graduate School of Education, May 1983.

156. Macdonald J: An investigation of body scheme in adults with cerebral vascular accident. Am J Occup Ther 14:72-79, 1960.

157. Magoun HW: The Waking Brain. Springfield, Illinois, Charles C Thomas Publ., 1969.

158. Mahoney J, Siev E: Provisional normative study of normal adults for Southern California figure ground, position in space and kinesthesia tests. Unpublished data, 1973.

159. Malkmus D: Integrating cognitive strategies into the physical therapy setting. Phys Ther 63(12):1952-1959, 1983.

160. Malec J, Questad K: Rehabilitation of memory after craniocerebral trauma: case report. Arch Phys Med Rehab 64:436-438, 1983.

161. Maloney MP, Payne L: Validity of the draw-a-person test as a measure of body image. Percept Motor Skills 29:119-122, 1969.

162. Massey EW, Coffey CE: Frontal lobe personality syndromes: ominous sequelae of head trauma. Postgrad Med 73(5):99-106, 1983.

163. Mayer-Gross W: Some observations of apraxia. Proc Roy Soc Med 28:1203-1212, 1934-1935.

164. McCollough NC III, Sarniento A: Functional prognosis of the hemiplegic. J Florida Med Assoc 57:31-34, 1970.

165. McFie J: The diagnostic significance of disorders of higher nervous activity. In Vinken PJ, Bruyn GW (eds.): Handbook of Neurophysiology. New York, American Elsevier Publishing Co., 1969, Vol. 4, pp. 1-11.

166. McFie J, Piercy MF, Zangwill OL: Visual spatial agnosias associated with lesions of the right cerebral hemisphere. Brain 73:167-189, 1950.

167. McFie J, Zangwill OL: Visual-constructive disabilities associated with lesions of the left cerebral hemisphere. Brain 83:243-259, 1960.

168. McWilliams P: Personal Computers and the Disabled. New York, Quantum Press, Doubleday & Co., 1984.

169. Meer B, Baker J: Reliability of measurements of intellectual functioning of geriatric patients. J Gerontol 20:110-114, 1965.

170. Meltzer M: Poor memory: a case report. J Clin Psychol 39(1):3-10, 1983.

171. Norman DA: What have the animal experiments taught us about human memory? In Deutsch JA (ed.): The Physiological Basis of Memory. New York, Academic Press, Inc.,1973.

172. Milner D: Use of microcomputers in the treatment of patients with physical disabilities. Phys Disab Spec Inter Sect Newsletter, 7(2):1, 1984.

158

173. Milner P: Physiological Psychology. New York, Holt, Rinehart and Winston, Inc., 1970.

174. Moffat N: Strategies of memory therapy. In Wilson BA, Moffat N (eds.): Clinical Management of Memory Problems. Rockville, Maryland, Aspen Publishers, 1984.

175. Moskowitz E, Lightbody EEH, Freitag NS: Long term follow-up of the post stroke patient. Arch Phys Med Rehab 53:167-172, 1972.

176. Mountcastle VB: The view from within: pathways to the study of perception. Johns Hopkins Med J 136:109-131, 1975.

177. Murrell FH: The effect of extensive practice on age difference in reaction time. J Gerontol 25:268-274, 1970.

178. Neles R: Verbal pictorial recording in the elderly. J Gerontol 31:421-427, 1976.

179. Ordy JM, Brizzee KR: Sensory coding: sensation perception, information processing, and sensory-motor integration from maturity to old age. In Ordy JM, Bizzee KR (eds.): Aging. Vol. 10. Sensory Systems and Communication in the Elderly. New York, Raven Press, 1979.

180. Ordy JM, Brizzee KR, Beavers T, Medart P: Age differences in the functional and structural organization of the auditory system in man. In Ordy JM, Brizzee KR (eds.): Aging. Vol. 10. Sensory Systems and Communication in the Elderly. New York, Raven Press, 1979.

181. Parente F: Cognitive rehabilitation and the use of computers. Paper presented to Baltimore Adult Communications Disorders Interest Group.

182. Parente F, Anderson JK: Techniques for improving cognitive rehabilitation: teaching organization and encoding skills. Cognit Rehabil 20-22, 1983.

183. Pascal GK, Suttell B: The Bender-Gestalt Test—Its Quantification and Validity for Adults. New York, Grune & Stratton, Inc., 1951.

184. Pasik P, Pasik T: Ocular movements in split brain monkeys. Adv Neurol 18:125-135, 1977.

185. Patterson KE, Baddeley AD: When face recognition fails. J Exp Psychol Hum Learn Mem 3:406-417, 1977.

186. Pehoski C: Analysis of perceptual dysfunction and dressing in adult hemiplegics. Thesis, Sargent College, Boston University, 1970.

187. Piasetsky E, Ben-Yishay Y, Weinberg J: The systematic remediation of specific disorders: selected application of methods derived in a clinical research setting. In Trexler LE (ed.): Cognitive Rehabilitation Conceptualization and Intervention. New York, Plenum Press, 1982.

188. Pickett JM, Bergman M, Levitt H: Aging and speech understanding. In Ordy JM, Bizzee KR (eds.): Aging. Vol. 10. Sensory Systems and Communication in the Elderly. New York, Raven Press, 1979.

189. Piercy M, Hecaen H, de Ajuriaguerra J: Constructional apraxia associated with unilateral cerebral lesions: left and right sided cases compared. Brain 83:225-242, 1960.

190. Pigott R, Brickett F: Visual neglect. Am J Nurs 66:101-105, 1966.

191. Podolsky S, Schachar R: Clinical manifestations of diabetic retinopathy and other diseases of the eye in the elderly. In Ordy JM, Bizzee KR (eds.): Aging. Vol. 10. Sensory Systems and Communication in the Elderly. New York, Raven Press, 1979.

192. Poon L, Fozard J: Speed of retrieval from long term memory in relation to age, familiarity, datedness of information. J Gerontol 33(5):711-717, 1978.

193. Rabbit P: Changes in problem solving ability in old age. In Birren J, Schaie K (eds.): Handbook of Psychology of Aging. New York, Von Nostrand Reinhold Co., 1977.

194. Rahmani L: The intellectual rehabilitation of brain-damaged patients. Clin Neuropsychol 4:44-45, 1982.

195. Rao S, Bieliauskas L: Cognitive rehabilitation two and one-half years post right temporal lobectomy. J Clin Neuropsychol 5(4):313-320, 1983.

196. Restak R: The Brain. Toronto, Bantam Books, 1984.

197. Riege W, Inman V: Age differences in nonverbal memory tasks. J Gerontol 36(1):51-58, 1979.

198. Riege WH, Klane LT, Metter EJ, Hanson WR: Decision speed and bias after unilateral stroke. Cortex 18:345-355, 1982.

199. Robins M, Baum H: Incidence. Part II. Stroke 12(2):45-58, 1981.

200. Rosensweig MR: Environmental complexity, cerebral change and behavior. Am Psychol 21:321-332, 1966.

201. Rothi L, Horner J: Restitution and substitution: two theories of recovery with application to neurobehavioral treatment. J Clin Neuropsychol 5(1):73-81, 1983.

202. Sarno J: Cerebral vascular diseases in the elderly: rehabilitation. In Albert M (ed.): Clinical Neurology of Aging. New York, Oxford University Press, 1984.

203. Sauguet J, Benton AL, Hecaen H: Disturbances of the body scheme in relation to language impairment and hemispheric locus of lesion. J Neurol Neurosurg Psychiat 34:496-501, 1971.

204. Sawtell R, Martin G: Perceptual problems of the hemiplegic patient. Lancet 87:193-196, 1967.

205. Schiffrin RM, Schneider W: Controlled and automatic human information processing. II. Perceptual learning, automatic attending, and a general theory. Psychol Rev 84:127-190, 1970.

206. Schonfield D: Translations in gerontology—from lab to life: utilizing information. Am Psychol 29:796-801, 1974.

207. Schwartz MT: New insights into vision development. J Optom Vis Devel 6(1):37-44, 1975.

208. Schwartz R, Shipkin D, Cermak L: Verbal and nonverbal memory abilities of adult brain-damaged patients. Am J Occup Ther 33(2):79-83, 1979.

209. Searleman A: A review of right hemisphere linguistic capabilities. Psychol Bull 84:503-528, 1977.

210. Seiderman A, Schneider S: The Athletic Eye. New York, Hearst Books, 1983.

211. Selecki BR, Herron JT: Disturbances of the verbal body image: a particular syndrome of sensory aphasia. J Nerv Ment Dis 141:42-51, 1965.

212. Sivak M, Hill C, Olson P: Computerized Video Tasks as Training Techniques for Driving-Related Perceptual Deficits of Persons with Brain Damage: A Pilot Evaluation. Ann Arbor, University of Michigan Transportation Research Institute, 1983.

213. Skilleck C: Computer assistance in the management of memory and cognitive impairment. In Wilson BA, Moffat N (eds.): Clinical Management of Memory Problems. Rockville, Maryland, Aspen Publishers, 1984.

214. Smith C: Computer update: special education. T.W.A. Ambassador, 86-87, June 1984.

215. Solet JM: Solet test for apraxia. Thesis, Boston University, 1974.

216. Solomon P, et al.: Sensory Deprivation. Cambridge, Harvard University Press, 1961.

217. Sperry R, Gazzaniga M: Language following surgical disconnection of the hemispheres. In Brain Mechanisms Underlying Speech and Language. New York, Grune & Stratton, Inc., 1967.

218. Stanley K: Survey conducted by St. Joseph Hospital, Albuquerque, New Mexico, 1984.

219. Stroop JR: Studies of interference in serial verbal reactions. J Exp Psychol 18:643-662, 1935.

220. Strub RL, Black FW: The Mental Status Examination in Neurology. Philadelphia, F.A. Davis Co., 1977.

221. Taylor MM: Analysis of dysfunction in the left hemiplegia following stroke. Am J Occup Ther 22:512-520, 1968.

222. Taylor MM: Controlled evaluation of percept-concept—motor training therapy after stroke resulting in left hemiplegia. Research grant RD-2215-M, sponsored by Rehabilitation Institute, Detroit, September 1969.

223. Travis LE (ed.): Handbook of Speech Pathology and Audiology. New York, Appleton-Century-Crofts, 1971.

224. Trombley C, Scott A: Occupational Therapy for Physical Dysfunction. Baltimore, The Williams & Wilkins Company, 1977.

225. Ullman M: Disorder of body image after stroke. Am J Nurs 64:89-91, 1964.

226. Vaughan WJ, Smitz P, Fatt I: The human lens—a model system for the study of aging. In Ordy JM, Bizzee KR (eds.): Aging. Vol. 10. Sensory Systems and Communication in the Elderly. New York, Raven Press, 1979.

227. Vinograd A, Taylor E, Grossman S: Sensory retraining of the hemiplegic hand. Am J Occup Ther 16:246-250, 1962.

228. Wall N, et al.: Hemiplegic Evaluation. Boston, Massachusetts Rehabilitation Hospital, 1979.

229. Warrington EK, James M: Disorders of visual perception in patients with localized cerebral lesions. Neuropsychologia 5:253-266, 1967.

230. Warrington EK, James M: An experimental investigation of facial recognition in patients with unilateral cerebral lesions. Cortex 3:317-327, 1967.

231. Warrington E, Rabin P: Visual span of apprehension in patients with unilateral cerebral lesions. Quart J Exp Psychol 23:423-431, 1971.

232. Weber MP: About this issue. Phys Disab Spec Inter Sect Newsletter 2(2):1, 1984.

233. Webser J, Scott R: The effects of self-instructional training on attentional deficits following head injury. Clin Neuropsychol 5:69-74, 1983.

234. Wechsler D: A standardized memory scale for clinical use. J Psychol 19:87-95, 1945.

235. Wechsler D: Manual for the Wechsler Adult Intelligence Scale. New York, The Psychology Corporation, 1955.

236. Weinberg J, Diller L, Gordon W, Gerstman L, Lieberman A, Lakin P, Hodges G, Ezrachi O: Visual scanning training effect on reading-related tasks in acquired right brain damage. Arch Phys Med Rehabil 58:479-486, 1977.

237. Weinberg J, Piasetsky E, Diller L, Gordon W: Treating perceptual organization deficits in non-neglecting right brain damage stroke patients. J Clin Neuropsychol 4(1):59-75, 1982.

238. Williams N: Correlations between copying ability and dressing activities in hemiplegia. Am J Phys Med 46:1332-1340, 1967.

239. Wilson B: Memory therapy in practice. In Wilson BA, Moffat N (eds.): Clinical Management of Memory Problems. Rockville, Maryland, Aspen Publishers, 1984.

240. Wilson B: Success and failure in memory training following a cerebral vascular accident. Cortex 18:581-594, 1982.

241. Wilson PG: Software selection and use in language and cognitive retraining. Cogn Rehab 1(1):9-10, 1983.

242. Wood RL: Management of attention disorders following brain injury. In Wilson BA, Moffat N (eds.): Clinical Management of Memory Problems. Rockville, Maryland, Aspen Publishers, 1984.

243. Young F: Early Experience and Visual Information Processing in Perceptual and Reading Disorders. Washington, D.C., National Academy of Sciences, 1970.

244. Young GC, Collens D, Hren M: Effect of pairing scanning training with block design training in the remediation of perceptual problems in left hemiplegics. J Clin Neuropsychol 5(3):201-212, 1983.

245. Young M: Problem-solving performance in two age groups. J Gerontol 21:505-509, 1966.

246. Zihl J, Von Cramon D: Restitution of visual function in patients with cerebral blindness. J Neurol Neurosurg Psychiat 42:312-322, 1979.

247. Zoltan B, Jabri J, Panikoff L, Ryckman D: Perceptual Motor Evaluation for Head Injured and Other Neurologically Impaired Adults. San Jose, Santa Clara Valley Medical Center, Occupational Therapy Department, 1983.

248. Zoltan B, Ryckman D: Head injury in adults. In Pedretti (ed.): Occupational Therapy for Physical Dysfunction (2nd edition). St. Louis, The C.V. Mosby Co., 1985.

Interviews:

249. Efferson, Laurie C., MS, OTR, Visual Retraining Specialist, San Francisco Bay Area, California.

250. Lemuel Shattuck Hospital, Occupational Therapy Staff.

251. Massachusetts Rehabilitation Institute, Louie Elfant, OTR.

252. New England Medical Center, Harriet N. Gordon, OTR, and Noreen Coffey, OTR.

253. New England Rehabilitation Center, Occupational Therapy Staff.

254. Okey, R., Specialty resource person for computers for the AOTA Physical Disabilities Special Interest Section. Personal communication, October 1984.

255. Youville Hospital, Occupational Therapy Staff.

Appendix A

Summary of Interitem Correlation Coefficients Praxis

Item	Match	Glass	Teeth	Paper	Ball	Fist	Salute	Pray	Wash	Boxer
Match	—									
Glass	0.61944	—								
Teeth	0.58051	0.95027	—							
Paper	0.84426	0.86180	0.78545	—						
Ball	0.95448	0.59676	0.63892	0.78089	—					
Fist	0.58849	0.90358	0.94711	0.75832	0.68825	—				
Salute	0.61500	0.93986	0.93109	0.80696	0.67207	0.98619	—			
Pray	0.95448	0.59676	0.63892	0.78089	1.00000	0.68825	0.67207	—		
Wash	0.53531	0.84296	0.79484	0.71500	0.55729	0.85320	0.88651	0.55729	—	
Boxer	0.55678	0.83547	0.63892	0.78089	0.44444	0.68825	0.79888	0.44444	0.78475	—

Appendix B

Computer Applications for Cognition and Language Skills

Peggy B. Wilson

The following is an annotated bibliography of hardware and software for the Apple II+ and IIe. I have found these programs or parts of the programs useful in various ways in working with neurologically impaired adults and children and in developing new programs. These comments are not meant to be endorsements of the products. If you are considering purchase of any computer product, you should see it before making a decision or ordering it "on approval." The prices given are retail list prices, but often discounts are available. When the product is not easily available commercially, I have listed the address. You are welcome to make copies of this list.

Hardware

Adaptive Firmware Card, Adaptive Peripherals, 4529 Bagley Ave. North, Seattle, WA 98103, (206) 633-2610, $300-$350. This is an important piece of hardware, which allows the user a great deal of flexibility in adapting software to the capabilities of the handicapped learner. Key features include the ability to slow the presentation speed of any program, to use a number of adaptive input devices such as microswitches or the large Unicorn keyboard, and to set up scanning procedures so that programs can be run without using the keyboard or in addition to the keyboard. It will also interface with the Echo II Speech Synthesizer and the Unicorn Keyboard.

Unicorn Keyboard, Unicorn Engineering Company, 6201 Harwood Ave., Oakland, CA 94618, (415) 428-1626, approximately $250. This large pressure sensitive membrane keyboard can be used as a lap communication board. It works through the Adaptive Firmware Card and can be programed to use virtually any program.

This appendix is reproduced with permission from Peggy B. Wilson, M.A., C.C.C., San Francisco State University, 1985.

Echo II Speech Synthesizer and *Textalker* software, Street Electronics, $135. This software has a card that fits into a slot in the computer and a speaker. It allows the user to type in words on the keyboard and have the synthesizer "say" the words. The Echo II can also be used with software from Laureate Learning Systems (1 Mill Street, Burlington, VT, [802] 862-7355) called *Speakup* ($95 - discount if buying Echo also), which already has the words included. Speakup has a vocabulary of 349 words and 40 functional phrases. Your own words can be added; however, this is time consuming. An additional 1500 word vocabulary is also available. As with all synthesized speech, it sounds rather mechanical. This may or may not be a problem for your clients.

Cassette Control Device, Hartley Software (vended by others as well), $79. This device allows you to use the computer to activate a cassette tape recorder. You can record any oral message you wish on the tape and synchronize it with the Hartley Create disks, such as *Create—Fill in the Blank* or *Create—Spell It,* $26.95 each. These allow the user to write lessons or tests with their speech recorded on the tape recorder but accommodates only 20 to 30 different items per tape.

Graphics Software and Hardware

The following can be used to create graphics and save them to a disk. The numerous applications of graphic screens include creating visuals for learners and capturing screens from other programs so that they can be studied or explained. Learners also like the idea of this electronic drawing. Once created and saved, these binary files can be interchanged and called up by other graphics programs. The pictures or results can also be printed by a dot matrix printer with the Grappler interface card or with Fontrix.

Koala Pad, Koala Technologies Corporation, Los Altos, CA, $129. This small graphics tablet (4 1/4 x 4 1/4 inch writing surface) uses MicroIllustrator software to permit the drawing of high resolution graphics on the screen. The Koala pad and scribe (or draw with your finger) can be used as an alternative input device for software using an Apple joystick. More educational software is being created for it as well. Atari and Commodore also sell their own versions of this device.

Flying Colors and slide projector, Computer Colorworks, Sausalito, CA, $39. This is software only, but it can be used on the Koala Pad or the user can draw with a joystick. It has more color combinations and a set of alphabet fonts so that the user can add text to a graph. The slide projector part allows the user to present a series of graphic frames at a specified interval or manually control presentation with arrow keys. *Flying Colors+* also has a print option ($69).

Power Pad, Chalk Board Inc., 3772 Pleasantdale Rd., Atlanta, GA, $89.

You also need the *Starter Kit for Apple Computer,* $49. This graphics tablet is larger (12 x 12 inch writing surface) but very similar to Koala. You may use the scribe or your finger to choose from the menu or to draw. The software is an enhanced version of MicroIllustrator, but it is not interchangeable with the two just mentioned. Because of its much larger surface and light weight, you may prefer it. Other educational software is being developed so that learners may use the pad as an input device in a learning task. IBM, Atari, and Commodore also sell versions of this software.

Fontrix, Data Transforms of Denver, CO, $75. This package allows the user to add a variety of sizes and styles of letters to the screen or graphic frames. The user may display on the screen or dump to a dot matrix printer. In addition, you may create a picture on one of the graphics programs and put your letters on it with Fontrix.

Print Shop, Broderbund, San Rafael, CA. This is less flexible but easier to use than Fontrix for creating printed cards, letterheads, or signs. It is menu driven through the process of creating the graphic.

Picture Writer, Scarborough Systems, $39. This is a graphics creation program like MicroIllustrator. Although it is slightly harder to use, it is forgiving and allows you to erase mistakes.

Pfs Graph, Software Publishing Corp., San Jose, CA, $128. This very simple graphics program will create and print bar and line graphs and pie charts. It will show in color on the screen. The user can create a master profile and then add or change data values for successive tests or other learners. It is quick and very user friendly, and the charts are impressive.

Fundamental Skills and Test Analysis

Foundations Package by Odie Bracy, Ph.D., available from Psychological Software Services, P.O. Box 29205, Indianapolis, Indiana 46229. This is a group of programs designed to work on basic cognitive functions such as attention, visual and auditory perception, and vigilance. Packages such as *Visuospatial* and *Memory* address additional fundamental skills at an expanded level. Whether this kind of training actually has generalizable effects has not been fully demonstrated, but initial results have been very promising. *Problem Solving* is a set of programs requiring analysis, deduction, and strategy at a very high level. For Apple and Atari, results go to screen, disk, or printer.

Sbordone-Hall Memory Battery by Robert Sbordone, Ph.D. This is a battery of tests that assesses various types of memory function.

WAIS-R Computer Report, WISC-R Computer Report, and *P.I.A.T. Error Analysis Report.* These programs are available from Southern Microsystems, P.O. Box 1981, Burlington, NC 27215, approximately $500 each. To run these programs, the user puts in the test scores and a seven or more page report is generated. The report includes detailed comparisons of the scores with various scales and statements of results. These comparisons can sometimes yield conflicting statements. The Woodcock-Johnson test was also accompanied by a scoring analysis program available from Sysdata for $495. A $59 version of this is available from the publishers of the test.

Language and Cognitive Tasks

Understanding Questions, $29, and *Understanding Stories,* $39, Sunset Software, Suite 414, 11750 Sunset Blvd., Los Angeles, CA 90049. These programs by speech and language pathologist Richard Katz, Ph.D., are helpful in differentiating question words and understanding information in short paragraphs. Performance data are printed out.

Crossword Magic, L & S Software, Box 70728, Sunnyvale, CA, $49.95. This classic piece of software creates a crossword puzzle as you type the words. Insert your own content and clues and it does the rest. It prints out beautifully on a dot matrix printer, or the user can play it on the computer. A good activity when working on categories or word association. Mildly to moderately involved users can create puzzles as well as work them.

Wordsearch and *Word Scramble,* Hi-Tech Software, Santa Cruz, CA, $24.95. This software allows the therapist to insert the words for which the computer will set up a search or scramble and then print out for the patient.

Computer Advanced Ideas, Berkeley, California, has four quiz show format programs that make it very easy for a therapist to use the format to write lessons and put in items on a particular content area or for a particular patient. These are *Tic Tac Show* (question-answer type), *Game Show* (word association task like "Password"), *Master Match* (like "Concentration"), and *Wizard of Words* (five word and spelling games). These cost $39.00 each and use high resolution graphic screens. The first two appeal to adults more.

Word Attack, Davidson Associates, Rancho Palos Verdes, CA, $49.95. This package offers a number of ways to learn vocabulary. It shows the learner the word, a synonym or descriptive phrase, and a sentence using the word. Next the learner can do a multiple choice task using the word or go on to fill in the blank in a sentence. It has a game format as a fifth option in which the learner matches definition and word. You can use one of the eight vocabulary levels in the program or add your own material. Data are presented as well as the items missed at the end of each section. *Math Master* is also available from the same publisher.

Missing Links (English Editor), Sunburst Communications, $59. In this software a passage is displayed with letters or words missing and the reader has to guess what they are. You can enter your own passages for your clients.

Alpine Skier, Data Command, Box 548, Kankakee, IL 60901. This contains four disks of three rounds with 12 sets, $29.00 per disk. It includes sets of reading exercises on "Fact and Opinion," "Cause and Effect," "Categorizing Words," and "Sentence Meaning." This is suitable for adults and children over 12. It keeps track of data on learner progress as well.

Early Words, Merry Bee Communications, $24. This software has several simple picture and word matching tasks. In addition it has a simple letter recognition task in which letters are rotated or printed in a different style and the patient is required to find the one that does not match. Reinforcement is juvenile.

Compu-Read, Eduware, $29.95. This software offers four tasks—letter matching, rapid word match, synonyms-antonyms, and sentence comprehension. The user has control of such parameters as length of display time, size of the letters in the display, number of trials, and increments by which the display time is increased or decreased. It has a lesson generator so that you can type in your items and thus control the content. Results are displayed in learner progress charts. The style is very structured and appeals to those who are "strictly business."

Story Machine, Spinnaker Software, $34.95. This software asks the learner to make sentences using a lexicon of about 50 words. The computer then shows an animated cartoon of the meaning expressed in the sentences. The learner must be able to use the keyboard, and spelling and grammar must be correct. The one drawback is that the program has several rules (such as only four actors on the screen) that disallow all of the possible combinations. Somewhat juvenile, but many adults enjoy it.

Story Tree, Scholastic Software, $49. This software is a writing program that allows the user to interact and write a story that actually offers branching in the plot. It appeals to ages 12 to adult. The creation part is similar to a combination of simple word processing and authoring. It can be used for more mildly involved patients who might be able to return to work.

Apple Logo. This software is easy to use, is interactive with the computer, and provides the user with generated text and graphics. Logo has important potential for handicapped individuals. It is easy to set up an individual lexicon of words and phrases or sentences so that a patient can find each word or phrase with a single key and thus communicate quickly on the screen or printer. He can string a number of these together for a conversation or letter. The HI program by "Kids Can Touch" is an introduction to Logo graphics that uses one key command to generate shapes on the screen.

Verb Viper (subject-verb agreement), *Spelling Wiz* (missing letter spelling), *Word Master* (synonym, antonym, and homonym), *Word Invasion* (classifying nouns, verbs, and so forth), and *Word Radar* (word matching and memory) are the language arts packages available from DLM, One DLM Park, P.O. Box 4000, Allen, TX 7500, (800) 527-4747, $44 each. They use an arcade game format with control for speed and difficulty. Word Master has been found very useful with adult aphasics. The program is creatively done and is fun for drill and practice. There are new disks with the same format that allow you to use the games but add your own content. These are Wiz Works, Mastermatch, and Alligator Alley. All include data and practice worksheets. There are math game formats as well (available from DLM) that also use the game formats.

Dragon's Keep, Sierra On-Line, $29, and *Lemonade,* Apple, are two simulations that involve a problem solving task in an adventure activity. Dragon involves reading, memory, and logical choices, and Lemonade requires some simple math. Reading is at the second grade level. Graphics and task appeal to kids.

Wordmaster, NTS Software, Rancho Palos Verde, CA. This software utilizes rhyming and word families to help the learner think of new words. Wordmaster also uses semantic cues to aid in word association. It is a very simple program and helpful with word recall.

Big Door Deal, Data Command, four disks, $29 each or $113 for the set. This game format consists of exercises using contextual clues, recognizing figurative language, completing analogies, and sequencing words or phrases in the correct order.

Grammar Problems for Practice, Milliken, $80 each set. These exercises include homonym, verb, and pronoun sets. They have pretests and mastery criteria and help screens as well. This can be used with patients with mild and moderate impairment in reading or grammar skills.

E-Z Learner, Silicon Valley Systems, $29. This is an easy drill format for you or your learner to write your own drills. The only problem is that it does require the learner to acknowledge an error when it is made.

Microzine Twistaplots, Scholastic Magazine, $39, or $129 for a one year subscription for four, for ages 10 and up. This reading task is a story offering the learner sets of choices as he goes through the adventure. Different choices lead to different events and consequences in the story. With an incredible amount of branching, it almost never ends the same way.

Visuospatial Tasks

See also *Visuospatial* and *Problem Solving* packages from Psychological Software Services listed on page 166.

Little Brickout from Apple Presents Apple II+ or Apple Sample Programs (usually free). This is a breakout game that starts off slowly and gets faster with successive hits.

Ribbit, Picadilly Software, Inc., is a slower version of Frogger. It is a visuospatial game in which the learner must first avoid and then seek out the objects that cross in front.

Perception, Eduware, Agourra, CA (D). This is a set of rather difficult perceptual tasks. When speed is an important factor, it can be slowed down using the Adaptive Firmware Card.

Apple Logo, Apple Computer Inc., Cupertino, CA, $150, and *HI* (Introduction to Logo Graphics) published by Kids Can Touch, 24 Beechwood Rd., Summit, NJ, $24.95. HI is used with Logo to create designs with shapes, colors, and line drawings on the screen. Each letter represents a shape.

Delta Drawing, Spinnaker Software, $59. This software can be used by high level learners to create drawings.

Facemaker, Spinnaker Software, $34.95. This is an electronic face building task with menus of eyes, noses, and so on like "Potato Head." The only negative factor is that part 3, the game, gives a "Bronx cheer" when the learner misses a sequence.

Squares, Trisensory Learning Co., Santa Cruz, CA, $39.95. This is a very simple block design task, appropriate for moderate to severe dysfunction.

Juggles Rainbow, published by The Learning Company, requires the learner to match the screen on various quadrants of the keyboard. Parts of the program are excellent; other parts are very juvenile.

Mastertype, Lightning Software, Box 11725, Palo Alto, CA, $39.95. This software has an exciting game format for training typing or word matching. Speed and difficulty level can be controlled easily. You may use any of the 17 lessons or create your own special ones. This program is used and enjoyed by all ages to increase skills with letters and words at the keyboard. Record keeping and parameter setting functions are excellent. Results can be printed out. While I am not advocating the teaching of typing or keyboarding skills, if the patient is going to use the keyboard rather than paddles, joy stick, or adaptive devices, some familiarity with the keyboard is needed. Since the learner has to attend to stimuli in the peripheral parts of the four quadrants, a scanning strategy must be developed.

Preschool IQ Builder (Part 1), Program Design Incorporated. This software has six programs that require the client to respond regardless of whether the items are the same or different. It starts with color and shape matching and progresses on to letters. Reinforcement is somewhat juvenile.

Spotlight, Children's Television Network, $39. This software is for ages 9 to adult and requires the learner to estimate an angle and bounce a beam of light to locate various targets.

Minnesota Educational Computer Consortium (MECC) has many different series of disks in elementary and secondary curriculum areas such as math, language arts, and sciences. They are generally good and the documentation is very important. They have some lesson creating capabilities as well.

Memory and Problem Solving

Einstein Memory Trainer, Einstein Corp., Los Angeles, $89. This package of programs is good for those with mild dysfunction. It systematically trains such strategies as visualization, association, and linking to increase memory abilities for names, faces, numbers, and word association. Learners can include some of their own items in parts of the tasks. For Apple and Atari.

Sbordone Memory Battery. See Fundamental Skills, page 166.

Memory Skills, Psychological Software Services (page 166). This set includes tests as well as visual, verbal, auditory, and spatial tasks. Some problem solving is required for the visual tasks. Dr. Bracy also has a Problem Solving set of programs, which involve deduction and strategy. See also MasterMatch from CAI, Word Radar from DLM, and Dragon's Keep under Language Skills.

Plato's Cave, Krell Software, $39. This is a multilevel problem solving task, which involves finding hidden markers and reflectors on the basis of the results obtained from shining a beam of light in a "cave." It is useful in structuring a sequence of problem solving tasks and can work well with the Spotlight program.

Speech Analysis

Voice Print by Peter Kosel is a public domain program that shows a spectrographic analysis of speech or other signals on the screen. The learner can compare his speech to a target utterance.

Survival Skills in the Community

Budgeting Tutorial and Budgeting Simulation, Computer Courseware Services (Division of EMC Publishing), 287 York Ave., St. Paul, MN 55101, (612) 771-1555, $55 each or $98 for both. These two programs have excellent content, graphics, and sequence. Real life problems are presented and choices are offered to the student.

You Can Bank on It, Computer Courseware Services, $325. This six disk program covers the essentials of banking transactions. Parts of it assume that the learner would now know why to use banks. Other parts are very good. Expensive and directed at special and vocational education.

Survival Math, Sunburst Publications, $50. This is a set of four simulations in which the learner has to carry out common tasks such as deciding the best value in a supermarket, managing resources in a hot dog stand, or planning a trip as a travel agent would. Math skills needed for each task are clearly specified.

Clinical Data Management

A number of programs can assist the clinician or therapist in efficiently maintaining clinical progress records, test results, and any background information. The following general types are described with their uses. If you are a user, you should analyze your needs and level of use before buying. The most expensive and most powerful programs may be more than you need and very cumbersome to learn and use.

Word Processing

The new word processing programs provide the possibility of faster and more efficient ways to compose reports with their electronic formating and editing modes. Most have a form fill-in capability that allows one to create a template type of report and fill in areas in which new information is required. The computer asks for information and automatically inserts your answer in the appropriate areas of the report. In this way you can fill in the blanks (such as a name or referral source) when that is called for, but you also have the flexibility of adding important information when it is needed to explain individual problems.

If you are going to use the computer yourself to create the document, a program that is powerful but easy to learn is advised. *Word Handler,* $59, and *Applewriter IIe,* $199, are very good. Easy but less powerful are *Bank Street Writer,* $69, and *Homeward,* $69, produced by Sierra On-Line.

Several creative clinicians have used word processing to create lessons for their patients. Dr. William Lynch has shown its actual use with an aphasic patient. One patient who has used an easy system remarked that it seemed even easier than writing!

Data Base Management

D-Base II (Ashton-Tate, $425 to $700) and *DB Master* (Stoneware Inc., $230) are the best known data management systems on microcomputers for clinics or small businesses. DB Master has a stat pak and two utilities disks ($100 each). Both are difficult to learn! They may be more than you need. If you are interested in very user friendly, easy packages to learn the basics, you might like *Data Factory* from Microlab ($180 to $300), *PFS* from Software Publishing Corp.($125), or *List Handler* from Silicon Valley Systems ($49). Briefly, all you do is to define the categories or "fields" in which you want to keep certain information, and the program will keep your data there and sort any record or field that you want. We have also used a simple data file manager to keep track of different kinds of items in a category as part of a divergent thinking task.

Electronic Spreadsheets

Programs such as *Visicalc* by Visicorp, and now the easier and more powerful *Multiplan* by Microsoft, can be used to keep, tabulate, and calculate any type of numerical data. You can use any formula to carry out these numerical analyses. You create each spreadsheet or template and it will tell you the results.

Grade Book is a system that will keep all your patient's scores and total, average rank, and sort them either by activity or by the student's name. It will generate a roster of the whole group or a detailed record for one student ($39.95). It's a real time saver.

Learning to Use the Computer

Apple Presents Apple (or How to Use the Keyboard), produced by Apple Computer (usually free), introduces the user to the Apple Computer keyboard functions. This is very good for the novice, those with computer phobias, or anyone unfamiliar with the functions and control keys of the Apple computer. This program is carefully sequenced and has prompts and informative feedback to guide the patient in the use of the computer. It is better for higher level patients.

Know Your Apple, Muse Software, $29.95. This program uses high resolution graphics and text to teach the user about the keyboard, the back and inside (including motherboard) of the computer, and the monitor and disk drive. This program is not as simple as the foregoing one, but it covers more ground. This program is perhaps more useful for the clinician than for the patient.

Appendix C

LESION SITES

The following illustrates the brain divisions as well as the vascular supply and lesion areas for certain perceptual deficits.

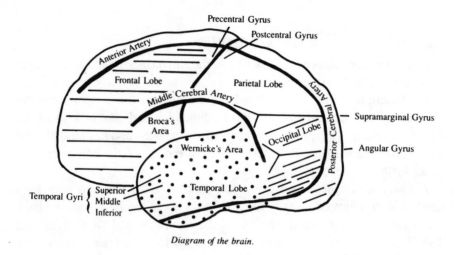

Diagram of the brain.

LESION SITES

Lobe and Vascular Supply*	Dominant Hemisphere (Left) Deficits	Nondominant Hemisphere (Right) Deficits
Frontal lobe vascular supply:	Expressive aphasia	Motor amusia
1. Internal carotid artery	Agraphia	Motor apraxia
2. Middle cerebral artery	Verbal apraxia	
3. Anterior cerebral artery	Motor apraxia	
Temporal lobe vascular supply:	Sensory amusia	Sensory amusia
	Receptive aphasia	Metamorphosia
1. Internal carotid artery	Auditory agnosia (rarely)	Constructional apraxia
2. Posterior cerebral artery	Alexia	
3. Middle cerebral artery	Agraphia	
	Associated with disorders of parietal lobe: apraxias, somatognosia, and acalculia	
Occipital lobe vascular supply:	Right hemianopsia	Prosopagnosia
	Alexia	Alexia
1. Posterior cerebral artery	Color agnosia	Color agnosia
	Receptive dysphasia	Dysgraphia
	Dyscalculia	Topographical disorientation
	Constructional apraxia	Dressing apraxia
	Simultanognosia	Visual object agnosia
	Visual object agnosia	Apractognosia
		Left hemianopsia
Parietal lobe vascular supply:	Tactile agnosia	Tactile agnosia
1. Internal carotid artery	Constructional apraxia	Constructional apraxia
2. Anterior cerebral artery	Visual object agnosia	Visual object agnosia
3. Posterior cerebral artery	Visual spatial agnosia	Visual spatial agnosia
4. Middle cerebral artery	Agraphia	Agraphia (possibly)
	Acalculia	Acalculia (possibly)
	Right/left discrimination	Right/left discrimination (possibly)
	Finger agnosia	
	Gerstmann's syndrome	Apractognosia
	Somatognosia	Amorphosynthesis
	Asymbolia	Unilateral neglect
	Ideomotor apraxia	Dressing apraxia
	Ideational apraxia	Prosopagnosia
	Simultanognosia	Topographical disorientation
		Anosognosia
		Alexia (possibly)
		Spatial relations syndrome

*References especially helpful for lesion sites and vascular supply are 60, 100, and 165.

The foregoing table classifies the perceptual deficits discussed in this manual by lesion sites for dominant and nondominant cerebral hemispheres with the corresponding vascular supply. The reader should remember that lesion sites widely vary from patient to patient and that this chart proposes only to represent the more common lesion sites described for various deficits.

Appendix D

FURTHER RESEARCH

Research concerning perceptual and cognitive problems for the adult hemiplegic is still in its beginning stages. Even though the perceptual and cognitive deficts and their corresponding lesion sites have often been described in literature, the clinician is more concerned with knowing how the existence of these problems relates to functional rehabilitation for the patient. With hospital stays averaging 30 to 90 days for the majority of hemiplegic patients in a rehabilitation setting, standardized testing with scores related to functional levels of activities of daily living and successful treatment techniques are crucial.

Currently there are few standardized perceptual and cognitive tests geared especially for the adult patient. Thus, in reviewing one patient's scores on the tests included here, one cannot compare scores with those of another patient, or draw any certain conclusions from the scores themselves. More important, in terms of validity, it is not known whether some of these tests actually evaluate what they purport to evaluate. Additionally, most test scores have not been conclusively related to specific functional skills, although a few studies have shown positive correlations between test scores and certain skills. Such information would be important when counseling the patient and family prior to discharging the patient.

At this point, it is also unknown whether perceptual and cognitive training for the adult stroke patient results in any learning, e.g., new memory patterns to replace those lost or damaged by the insult. If learning does occur, either in perceptual or cognitive areas alone or generalized to basic functional skills, the question of which training approach or combination of approaches proves most successful, becomes exceedingly important. Other areas for future research also arise: Does learning occur in patients with brain damage in either hemisphere, or in one more than in the other? If perceptual and cognitive skills are relearned, how long a time period is necessary and can the patient continue to improve his skills as long as he receives various treatments?

There are still areas in the realm of perceptual and cognitive deficit descriptions and occurrences that need additional research. However, for occupational therapists to perform more effectively in helping stroke patients to regain independence, they need valid, reliable evaluation and treatment techniques for such patients. We encourage every therapist to use all or any of the foregoing material for research ideas. The references beginning on page 151 are a good source for beginning data. For those interested in designing their own experimental studies, we would suggest any good book on behavioral research to aid in the correct procedures for stating hypotheses, selecting samples, and delineating methods.

One good reference is *Foundations of Behavioral Research* by Fred N. Kerlinger, New York, Holt, Rinehart and Winston Inc., 1964.

Appendix E

GLOSSARY

Abstraction: the ability to think conceptually.

Acalculia, dyscalculia:* a disturbance in the ability to solve simple or complex mathematical problems.

Agnosia: the failure to recognize familiar objects perceived by the senses.

Agrammatism: the inability to arrange words in grammatical sequence or to form an intelligible sentence.

Agraphia, dysgraphia:* a disturbance in writing intelligible words.

Ahylognosia: the inability to differentiate qualities of materials.

Alexia, dyslexia:* a difficulty in reading.

Amusia: a defect in auditory perception involving perception of music.

Anomia: the inability to remember and express names (nouns) of persons and objects.

Anosodiaphoria: one's unconcern for his paralysis.

Anosognosia: a severe form of neglect such that the patient fails to recognize his paralysis.

Aphasia, dysphasia:* inability to express oneself through speech or the inability to comprehend the spoken word.

Aphemia: the inability to express oneself in words, i.e., expressive aphasia.

Apractognosia: consists of several different apraxic and agnostic syndromes, all derived from an impairment of spatial perspective.

Apraxia: the inability to perform certain purposeful movements without the loss of motor power, sensation, or coordination.

Astereognosis: see TACTILE AGNOSIA.

Asymbolia: the inability to comprehend and use words, gestures, or any type of symbols.

Attention: an active process that helps to determine which sensations and experiences are alerting and relevant to the individual.

Auditory agnosia: the inability to recognize differences in sounds.

Autotopagnosia: an impairment in the recognition of body parts.

Body image: one's mental representation of his body that expresses one's feelings and thoughts about one's body rather than representing an exact picture of the physical structure.

---

* The prefixes "a," meaning totally without, and "dys," meaning impairment of, are often used interchangeably when referring to these deficits.

Body scheme: a postural model one has of himself, having to do with how one perceives the position of the body and the relationship of body parts. It is believed to be the basis for all motions.

Cognition: includes the processes of knowing and understanding, awareness, judgment, and decision making.[65]

Color agnosia: the inability to recognize differences in color.

Constructional apraxia: the inability to produce designs in two or three dimensions, by copying, drawing, or constructing, upon command or spontaneously.

Dressing apraxia: the inability to dress oneself because of a disorder in body scheme or motor planning.

Expressive aphasia: the inability to express oneself in words.

Figure ground: the ability to distinguish the foreground from the background.

Finger agnosia: doubt and hesitation concerning the fingers.

Form constancy: the ability to attend to subtle variations in form.

Gerstmann's syndrome: a syndrome believed to be derived from a lesion in the dominant hemisphere involving the following symptoms: dysgraphia, dyscalculia, finger agnosia, and right/left discrimination.

Hemianopsia: blindness for one half of the field of vision in one or both eyes.

Homonymous hemianopsia: blindness of right sided or left sided fields of both eyes.

Ideational apraxia: the inability to carry out activities automatically or on command because the patient no longer understands the concept of the act.

Ideomotor apraxia: the inability to imitate gestures or perform a purposeful motor task on command even though the patient fully understands the idea or concept of the task.

Initiation: the ability to start a task; impaired initiation may appear as decreased spontaneity, decreased productivity, slowness of response, or lost initiative.

Macrosomatognosia: a disorder in body scheme that distorts one's perception of his body as abnormally large.

Memory: perception that has been stored at an earlier time that can then be brought forward; a dynamic process involving many associated components. Memory types include recognition, iconic, short term, semantic, and long term. For a detailed definition of these and related memory terms, the reader is referred to Figure 8-1.

Mental inflexibility: associated with stimulus-bound, perseverative behavior; difficulty with association ability and the ability to generalize knowledge for future problem solution.

Metamorphopsia: a visual distortion of objects although the object may be recognized accurately.

Microsomatognosia: a disorder in body scheme that distorts one's perception of his body as abnormally small.

Morphognosia: the inability to tactilely recognize two dimensional shapes with vision occluded.

Motor apraxia: loss of kinesthetic memory patterns so that purposeful movement cannot be achieved even though the idea and purpose of the task are understood.

Ocular pursuits: visual scanning.

Perception: the ability to interpret sensory messages from the internal and external environment such that the sensation has meaning.

Perseveration: continued repetition of a movement or word.

Planotopokinesia: a disorganization of discriminative spatial judgment.

Planning: the determination and organization of the steps needed to achieve a goal.

Position in space: the ability to understand and deal with concepts of spatial position, such as up-down, in-out, left-right, and before-behind.

Problem solving: involves the integration of attention to task, information access, organization, planning, and judgment; the ability to modify, transform, and organize information to generate a solution.

Prosopagnosia: the inability to recognize differences in faces.

Receptive aphasia: the inability to comprehend the spoken word.

Right/left discrimination: a deficit in understanding and using the concepts of right and left.

Saccadic eye movements: sequenced rapid eye movements; the ability to localize stimuli; involves peripheral vision.

Somatognosia: the unawareness of body structure and the failure to recognize one's parts and their relationship to each other.

Tactile agnosia: the inability to recognize objects or forms by touch although touch sensation is still intact.

Unilateral body agnosia: neglect of the left side of body.

Unilateral neglect: the inability to integrate and use perceptions from the left side of the body or the left side of the environment.

Unilateral spatial agnosia: neglect of the left side of visual space.

Verbal apraxia: difficulty in forming and organizing intelligible words although the musculature required to do so remains intact.

Visual attention: voluntary act of visual fixation; focused gaze.

Visual field: normal visual field approximately 60 degrees upward and 60 degrees inward, 70 to 75 degrees downward, and 100 to 110 degrees outward.[116]

Visual neglect: neglect of a portion of the visual field in addition to or in the absence of a visual field deficit.

Visual object agnosia: the inability to recognize objects, although visual acuity may or may not be intact.

Visual spatial agnosia: a deficit in perceiving spatial relationships between objects or between objects and self, independent of visual object agnosia.